Dear Reader,

My earliest food memories take me back to sitting around the kitchen table, having family-style dinners with my mom, dad, sister, and brother. We ate dinner together most nights, and my siblings and I were often involved in helping to prepare the meals—sautéing , setting the table, pouring glasses of milk. I loved to help in the kitchen as a child, and this **built the foundation** for me to be able to cook and take care of myself as an adult.

As I grew up and left the house, I realized that not everyone had the same experiences as me, and this fueled my passion to become a registered dietitian and help others **learn to cook** and take care of themselves. Now with a family of my own, it's important for me to teach my children the same skills I learned growing up—not only how to cook, but how to take care of themselves.

In this book, I share my knowledge about nutrition and how it can have a **profound impact** on our minds and bodies. It's my goal to teach others not to obsess over what we eat or how much we exercise, but instead to focus on the positives and learn what we can add to our lives rather than take away. I truly believe we can design a life where maintaining a healthy lifestyle is both rewarding and enjoyable.

Emily Weeks, RDN, LD

Welcome to the Everything® Series!

These handy, accessible books give you all you need to tackle a difficult project, gain a new hobby, comprehend a fascinating topic, prepare for an exam, or even brush up on something you learned back in school but have since forgotten.

You can choose to read an Everything® book from cover to cover or just pick out the information you want from our four useful boxes: Questions, Facts, Alerts, and Essentials. We give you everything you need to know on the subject, but throw in a lot of fun stuff along the way too.

question	fact
Answers to common questions.	Important snippets of information.

alert	essential
Urgent warnings.	Quick handy tips.

We now have more than 600 Everything® books in print, spanning such wide-ranging categories as cooking, health, parenting, personal finance, wedding planning, word puzzles, and so much more. When you're done reading them all, you can finally say you know Everything®!

PUBLISHER Karen Cooper

MANAGING EDITOR Lisa Laing

COPY CHIEF Casey Ebert

PRODUCTION EDITOR Jo-Anne Duhamel

ACQUISITIONS EDITOR Lisa Laing

SENIOR DEVELOPMENT EDITOR Lisa Laing

EVERYTHING® SERIES COVER DESIGNER Erin Alexander

THE
EVERYTHING®
EASY
ANTI-
INFLAMMATORY
COOKBOOK

EMILY WEEKS, RDN, LD

200 Recipes to Naturally Reduce Your Risk of Heart Disease, Diabetes, Arthritis, Dementia, and Other Inflammatory Diseases

ADAMS MEDIA
NEW YORK   LONDON   TORONTO   SYDNEY   NEW DELHI

To Nick, Abigail, & Harrison

Acknowledgments

Thank you to my friends and family for supporting and encouraging me through years of recipe testing and messy kitchens. To my parents, for instilling in me a love of food and cooking. To my sister Leslie, who inspired many of the plant-based recipes in this book. To my husband, Nick, who has stood by my side from the beginning of my journey through the world of recipe development and photography.

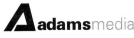

Adams Media
An Imprint of Simon & Schuster, Inc.
100 Technology Center Drive
Stoughton, Massachusetts 02072

An Everything® Series Book.

Everything® and everything.com® are registered trademarks of Simon & Schuster, Inc.

First Adams Media trade paperback edition December 2022

ADAMS MEDIA and colophon are trademarks of Simon & Schuster.

For information about special discounts for bulk purchases, please contact Simon & Schuster Special Sales at 1-866-506-1949 or business@simonandschuster.com.

The Simon & Schuster Speakers Bureau can bring authors to your live event. For more information or to book an event contact the Simon & Schuster Speakers Bureau at 1-866-248-3049 or visit our website at www.simonspeakers.com.

Interior layout by Kellie Emery
Interior photographs by Emily Weeks
Nutritional analysis by Mitali Shah-Bixby

Manufactured in the United States of America

1 2022

Library of Congress Cataloging-in-Publication Data has been applied for.

ISBN 978-1-5072-1989-8
ISBN 978-1-5072-1990-4

Many of the designations used by manufacturers and sellers to distinguish their products are claimed as trademarks. Where those designations appear in this book and Simon & Schuster, Inc., was aware of a trademark claim, the designations have been printed with initial capital letters.

Contains material adapted from the following title published by Adams Media, an Imprint of Simon & Schuster, Inc.: *The Everything® Anti-Inflammation Diet Book* by Karlyn Grimes, MS, RD, LDN, copyright © 2011, ISBN 978-1-4405-1029-8.

Contents

Introduction

From the first day of life and throughout the life cycle, the human body is constantly growing, changing, and healing. And every day, the body naturally responds to viruses, bacteria, toxins, and other damaging factors like cuts and scrapes by activating a natural inflammatory response.

However, sometimes this inflammatory response is not turned off after the threat is gone, leaving a form of "silent" inflammation that can damage the body. Instead of protecting and healing the body, inflammation becomes the enemy. Although inflammation is a natural and essential response to injury, irritation, and infection, there can be too much of a good thing. Heart disease, diabetes, cancer, Alzheimer's disease, and autoimmune diseases are all linked to uncontrolled inflammation.

Luckily, more and more research supports specific behaviors that can significantly reduce the presence of inflammation in the body. Rather than treat the problems linked to inflammation, the focus has turned to proactively preventing inflammation. Embracing an anti-inflammatory lifestyle can help treat or reduce the risk of a variety of chronic diseases and conditions. This includes choosing fruits and vegetables rich in phytochemicals and antioxidants, mostly plant-based protein foods, whole grains, healthy fats, and probiotics. Adequate sleep and fluids, exercise, stress reduction, and dietary supplements round out the anti-inflammatory menu.

Whether you're dealing with chronic inflammation or simply trying to avoid it in the first place, in this cookbook you'll find two hundred easy and satisfying recipes to make your transition to an anti-inflammatory lifestyle effortless. Start the day with a fruit-filled smoothie or a hearty "Sausage" Bread Pudding (Chapter 2). For lunch, choose from fresh salads like Quinoa Apple Salad (Chapter 6) or a cup of icy Gazpacho (Chapter 4). You'll also find lots of ideas for expanding your weeknight dinner options, from Crispy Tofu Tacos with Avocado Crema (Chapter 8) to Curried Red Lentils and Tomatoes (Chapter 10). And of course, there are healthy choices for dessert, including Dark Chocolate Cherry Cake with Ganache (Chapter 12), which only *sounds* decadent.

Along the way, *The Everything® Easy Anti-Inflammatory Cookbook* will teach you about foods that reduce inflammation and give you tips on adding them to your everyday meals. As you embark on this journey of healthier eating and habits, try not to focus on what you shouldn't eat. Think about the joy of discovering new foods and reimagined favorites as you provide your body with the fuel it needs to keep inflammation at bay. You'll be amazed at how good you'll feel!

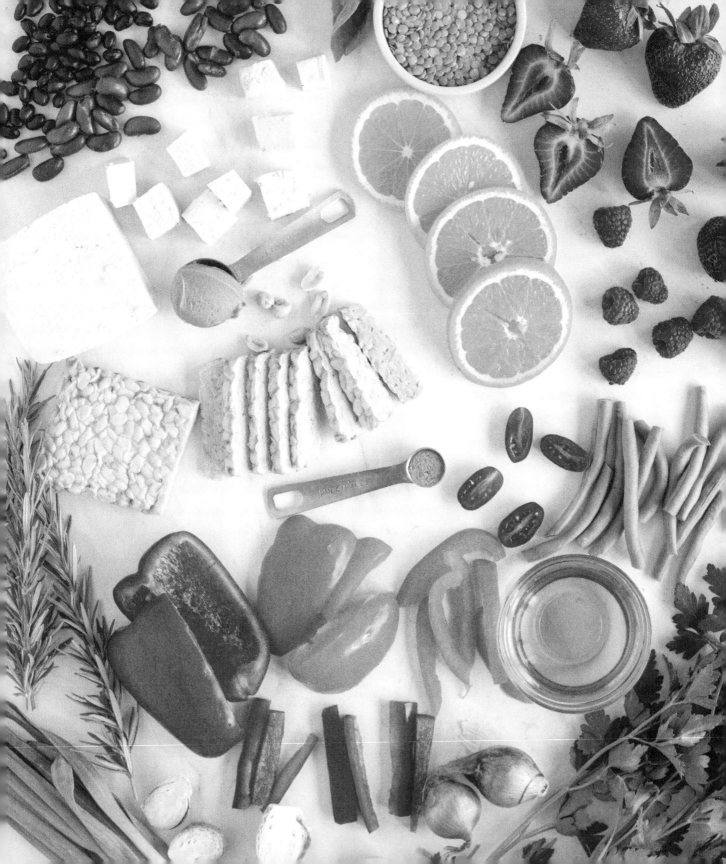

CHAPTER 1

The Anti-Inflammatory Lifestyle

The anti-inflammatory lifestyle isn't a fad diet. It's a lifestyle change that can add years to your life and can help treat or reduce the risk of a variety of chronic diseases and conditions. In this chapter, you'll learn about the roots of inflammation and how to build a healing lifestyle that can reduce inflammation for good. You'll learn how to build an anti-inflammatory plate with plenty of fruits, vegetables, whole grains, and plant-based proteins, especially the foods that are high in antioxidants and will become your new staples. You'll also find tips on day-to-day changes such as getting enough sleep, reducing stress, staying hydrated, and becoming physically active—all important parts of this healthy lifestyle. Overall, it's about making small, sustainable changes when you can, rather than undertaking an entire life makeover and striving for a perfect diet. Every small change you make contributes to lowering inflammation in the body and improving your quality of life. So let's get started!

Understanding the Inflammatory Response

Whenever you are exposed to an infectious agent or experience tissue injury or damage, your immune system mounts an inflammatory response. For example, when you cut your finger and it becomes red and swollen, inflammation is working its magic, and it's a lifesaver. During this response, your body releases pro-inflammatory chemicals and hormones that are equipped to deal with any threat to the body. These mercenaries attack unwelcome foreign invaders such as bacteria while tending to harmed tissue. Blood flow increases to places that require healing. Pain intensifies as a signal that something is wrong within the body.

fact

The body uses fatty acids to make eicosanoids. Omega-6 fatty acids produce the eicosanoids that promote inflammation and blood clotting, suppress the immune system, and reduce healthy high-density lipoprotein (HDL) cholesterol levels. Omega-3 fatty acids have the opposite effect of omega-6 fatty acids as a result of the eicosanoids they synthesize. So the more omega-3 fatty acids you consume, the more anti-inflammatory eicosanoid generation in your body.

The main hormones that control the inflammatory response are called eicosanoids, which include prostaglandins, prostacyclins, thromboxanes, and leukotrienes. Eicosanoids influence many of the bodily systems and processes. In addition to triggering inflammation, eicosanoids, most notably the prostaglandins, are what promote pain, fever, and blood clotting when an injury occurs in the body.

The inflammatory response is normal and is the cornerstone of the body's healing response. Under normal circumstances, once the threat is under control, anti-inflammatory substances are released to turn off the immune response.

The Overactive Immune System

Sometimes inflammation gets the upper hand and continues to operate chronically. This causes continual secretion of pro-inflammatory chemicals. Chronic release and circulation of these chemicals results in an attack on healthy cells, blood vessels, and tissues.

Damage to blood vessels can promote atherosclerosis, a process that results in narrowing of the arteries. If pancreatic tissue is harmed, type 2 diabetes can develop. Injury to joint tissue, when the immune system mistakenly attacks normal tissue, can contribute to autoimmune disorders such as arthritis. Pro-inflammatory chemicals can also alter normal brain chemistry and potentially contribute to dementia and Alzheimer's disease. Over time, chronic inflammation causes inflammatory chemicals to damage your body as you go about your normal daily activities.

Other diseases and conditions thought to be associated with chronic inflammation include, but are not limited to, allergies, anemia, cancer, congestive heart failure, fibromyalgia, kidney failure, lupus, pancreatitis, psoriasis, and stroke.

Free Radicals: Inflammation Activators

Chronic inflammation creates an environment that fosters free radical production. Free radicals are continually being produced in your cells, and a certain level of free radical production is completely normal, just like the little pockets of benign inflammation present throughout the body. When free radical production exceeds the body's natural ability to impede their production, however, extensive bodily damage occurs.

What Is a Free Radical?

Free radicals are chemicals that contain unpaired electrons. In nature, electrons like to exist in pairs. Since free radicals are missing an electron, they travel through the body looking for electrons to steal so they can become stable. Free radicals commonly steal electrons from polyunsaturated fats situated within the membranes of nearby cells. They also target DNA within the nucleus of the body's cells. Free radical alterations to the DNA code can lead to uncontrolled cell growth and cancer.

When free radicals steal electrons from other substances in the body, they cause these substances to also become free radicals. This leads to a chain reaction because each modified cell will try to become stable and steal from another vulnerable cell in the body.

Too many free radicals in the body can promote cancer growth, increase the risk of high blood pressure, and damage cells. In the long run, free radicals stimulate inflammation and thereby perpetuate the inflammatory cycle. Management of inflammation is essential for squelching free radicals before they can run rampant in the body.

Fortunately, there are numerous dietary and lifestyle anti-inflammatory options that can be followed to put out the flames of inflammation. Following an anti-inflammatory lifestyle will keep inflammation at bay and help resolve the symptoms of chronic diseases.

The Disease-Busting Benefits of an Anti-Inflammatory Lifestyle

Inflammation contributes to multiple chronic illnesses that are costly and can corrode your quality of life. If left to its own devices, inflammation can take its toll on the body over time without your even knowing it. It's essential to gain a better understanding of the disease-busting benefits of the anti-inflammatory lifestyle before inflammation gets the best of you.

Heart Disease

Certain lifestyle factors encourage the development of cardiovascular disease, such as a diet high in fat, sedentary behaviors, cigarette smoking, stress, and having chronically elevated blood pressure and cholesterol levels. Cutting back on red meat, high-fat dairy, trans and saturated fats, and processed carbohydrates while increasing consumption of fatty fish, colorful fruits and vegetables, and fiber-rich foods will inevitably lead to lower blood pressure, cholesterol, and inflammation in the body.

Cancer

Chronic inflammation creates an environment that fosters free radical production. These free radicals can cause damage to genetic material in healthy cells. As altered cells continue to grow and divide, cancerous tumors can occur. Although chronic inflammation and free radicals will not always initiate cancer, they can establish the ideal environment for cancer cells to thrive. An anti-inflammatory lifestyle can halt excessive free radical activity and reduce the risk of damaged cells reproducing uncontrollably.

Dementia and Alzheimer's Disease

Research has shown that chronic inflammation can destroy brain cells and attack nerve cells, both of which can contribute to dementia, Alzheimer's disease, and the cognitive and behavioral impairments evident during aging. Fortunately, you have ammunition in your food supply that can help reduce the incidence of Alzheimer's and dementia. A new study published in the journal *Neurology* indicates that people who consumed a greater amount of pro-inflammatory foods were associated with an increased risk of dementia and cognitive decline. The data suggests that participants in the study who tended to choose less processed, more nutrient-dense foods had a lower incidence of dementia. Other recent studies have shown that certain phytochemicals may stop free radicals from causing damage to brain cells. To maximize phytochemical intake, choose fruits and vegetables that make up the colors of the rainbow. Foods high in omega-3 fatty acids, such as fatty fish, can also be used as dietary reinforcements against Alzheimer's.

Diabetes

Insulin is a hormone that acts like a key to allow body cells to accept glucose to use for energy. As blood sugar levels increase, the pancreas makes more insulin to try to get cells to open, but eventually the pancreas can't make enough insulin to meet the body's demands. At the same time, muscle, fat, and liver cells become resistant to insulin and take in less sugar. Too much sugar circulating in the bloodstream can cause prediabetes and eventually type 2 diabetes. High blood sugar is damaging to the body, and it can cause inflammation, heart disease, and kidney disease. Lifestyle changes that can help to manage diabetes include becoming physically active and eating foods rich in omega-3 fatty acids, low-glycemic-index foods such as non-starchy or low-starch fruits and vegetables, and lean meats and low-fat dairy.

Autoimmune Diseases

Autoimmune disorders such as rheumatoid arthritis, inflammatory bowel diseases like Crohn's disease, lupus, and asthma occur when the body's immune system attacks its own cells. This turns on a systemic inflammatory response that can spur inflammation throughout the body.

---

alert

Most individuals, whether they are in the early stages of an autoimmune disorder or the later stages, have "flares"—or an exacerbation of their symptoms—when they are stressed out. Scheduling stress-free or stress-relieving activities such as meditation, yoga, walking, running, or any other type of activity that quiets your body is key to keeping your immune system calm, cool, and collected. It is surprising what a positive effect these activities can have on a flare-up.

A study published in *The Journal of Rheumatology* found that those individuals who cut back on foods high in saturated fat such as meat and high-fat dairy foods experienced less joint tenderness and swelling. A vegetarian diet may also help calm flares associated with autoimmune disorders.

The Bottom Line on Inflammation and Chronic Disease

The control of inflammation is absolutely essential if the prevalence of chronic diseases such as heart disease, cancer, Alzheimer's disease, diabetes, and autoimmune disorders is to be reversed. Cutting back on red meat, high-fat dairy, trans and saturated fats, and processed carbohydrates while increasing consumption of fatty fish, colorful fruits and vegetables, and fiber-rich foods will inevitably lead to a reduction in the risk of inflammation and related chronic diseases.

Building an Anti-Inflammatory Plate

You can extinguish the flames of chronic inflammation before they grow out of control. A combination of healthy fats, fruits and vegetables, lean proteins, and whole grains can help you nip inflammation in the bud and enjoy many disease-busting benefits.

Fruits and Vegetables

Fruits and vegetables are major storehouses of phytochemicals and antioxidants, both of which have anti-inflammatory powers. Plants rely on phytochemicals for their own protection and survival. These potent chemicals help plants resist the attacks of bacteria and fungi, the potential havoc brought on by free radicals, and the constant exposure to ultraviolet light from the sun. Fortunately, when we consume plants, their chemicals are infused into our bodies' tissues and provide ammunition against disease.

In a similar manner to phytochemicals, antioxidants halt and repair free radical damage throughout the body. The most potent antioxidants include vitamin A, vitamin C, vitamin E, and selenium. In addition to fruits and vegetables, these free radical squelchers inhabit whole grains, vegetable oils, nuts, and seeds.

Protein

Dietary protein is responsible for the growth, maintenance, and repair of the body, but it can also contribute to chronic disease development if not chosen properly and in the correct amounts. Fatty and processed meats and high-fat dairy items should be chosen less often. These high-protein foods are also high in inflammation-promoting saturated fats and cholesterol.

Lean meats, white-meat poultry, eggs, and low-fat milk, cheese, and yogurt, on the other hand, contain less of these pro-inflammatory fats. Cold-water fish offers plenty of quality protein with a kick of anti-inflammatory omega-3 fatty acids.

There is new research that shows eating primarily plant-based proteins, such as soy foods, beans, lentils, whole grains, seeds, and nuts, will further reduce the presence of pro-inflammatory agents in the body while giving you a blast of phytochemicals and antioxidants.

Whole Grains

Whole grains are high in fiber content and offer a significant contribution of vitamins, minerals, and phytochemicals. A whole grain consists of the fiber-rich bran, the germ, and the endosperm, in contrast to a refined grain, which contains only the endosperm (the starchiest part of the grain). The higher fiber content of whole grains slows the digestion of starch and reduces the speed at which nutrients empty from the stomach. Both of these processes prevent spikes in blood sugar levels, which helps in management of blood insulin levels. All these adjustments can ultimately prevent numerous chronic diseases such as diabetes, heart disease, and cancer.

Whole grains to consider include amaranth, barley, brown rice, buckwheat, couscous, millet, oatmeal, popcorn, and quinoa.

Anti-Inflammatory Fats

Saturated fats are nonessential fats commonly found in meats, high-fat dairy products, and eggs. Although these foods provide important vitamins and minerals, saturated fats can promote inflammation, which is demonstrated by their ability to increase the inflammatory biomarkers in the blood.

---

fact

Although chocolate is high in saturated fat, it also contains numerous beneficial compounds. For example, chocolate is rich in antioxidants that fight free radicals as well as anti-platelet factors that reduce the risk of unnecessary blood clotting. Dark chocolate has the highest concentration of these healthy phytochemicals. Choose dark chocolate that offers at least 65 percent cocoa content to maximize the phytochemical infusion.

In contrast, omega-3 fatty acids have an anti-inflammatory effect in the body. These fatty acids are converted into hormone-like substances called eicosanoids, which have the overall effect of dilating blood vessels, minimizing blood clotting, and reducing inflammation. To increase your consumption of omega-3 fatty acids, try to eat fatty fish two to three times per week. The top fish choices include cold-water fish such as albacore tuna, anchovies, Atlantic herring, halibut, lake trout, mackerel, sardines, striped sea bass, and wild salmon.

Even though fish is your best option since it offers the most omega-3 bang for your buck, there are alternatives. The plant version of omega-3 fatty acids is alpha-linolenic acid (ALA), which can be converted into anti-inflammatory eicosanoids. ALA intake can be increased by using canola and flaxseed oils; adding ground flaxseed to salads, cereal, and other dishes; snacking on walnuts; choosing eggs from chickens fed grains rich in omega-3s; and eating foods rich in soy such as soybeans and tofu.

---

essential

Studies have confirmed that monounsaturated fats are anti-inflammatory fats as well, and olive oil is at the top of the list. The polyphenols in olive oil protect the heart and blood vessels from inflammation. Other healthy foods high in monounsaturated fats include peanut and canola oils, avocados, and nuts such as peanuts, walnuts, almonds, and pistachios. These foods are a delicious and satisfying way to take the wind out of the sails of inflammation.

Unfortunately, the body is not very efficient at converting ALA into eicosanoids. You need to consume three to four times as much ALA from plant-based foods to equal the amount found in a 3-ounce serving of fish. If you don't eat fish, you should consider taking a daily fish oil supplement.

Probiotics and Prebiotics

All humans have millions and millions of naturally occurring bacteria in their bodies. Normally, bacteria get a bad rap, but the right types of bacteria, specifically *Lactobacillus* and *Bifidobacterium*, can keep you healthy and even prevent disease. They support the immune system, keeping it strong and better able to fend off disease and illness. Ideally, your bowels contain about 85 percent "good" bacteria and only about 15 percent "bad" bacteria, but modern life has thrown off this balance for many Americans. The processed food supply and the overuse of antibiotics have reduced the colonies of good bacteria in the gut, but thankfully there is a solution.

You can help good bacteria flourish by consuming foods that contain high concentrations of healthy probiotics, such as *Lactobacillus acidophilus*. Fermented milk products such as yogurt, kefir, and some soy-based beverages will increase the probiotic bacteria within your body. Look on the label for the statement "live and active cultures" to ensure that you are increasing your consumption of probiotics. Miso, a Japanese condiment consisting of fermented soybean paste, can also augment beneficial bacteria.

It's also beneficial to increase your intake of prebiotics. Prebiotics are the nondigestible nutrients, primarily soluble fibers, that are used as an energy source by the bacteria (probiotics) that live in your intestines. Foods such as whole grains, onions, bananas, garlic, artichokes, and flaxseeds naturally contain prebiotics; you can also find them in a variety of fortified foods, beverages, and dietary supplements.

Supplements, Herbs, and Spices

Over the years, numerous dietary supplements, spices, and herbs have been found to have beneficial anti-inflammatory effects. Many of these substances can be incorporated into your diet without much effort and offer huge paybacks.

Vitamin D

Recent research has found that 75 percent of Americans are not receiving the recommended amounts of vitamin D. The resulting deficiency can have a negative impact on the immune system, which can increase the risk of developing hypertension, heart disease, diabetes, cancer, and a variety of autoimmune conditions.

Because there are only a few natural food sources of vitamin D, including fatty fish, fish oils, and fortified milk, alternate sources of vitamin D appear essential to satisfy current recommendations. Consuming fatty fish at least two times per week will not only boost your vitamin D intake but will provide your body with heart-healthy, inflammation-busting omega-3 fats as well. In addition to a variety of vitamin D–fortified foods, aim for two to three servings of vitamin D–fortified milk, yogurt, or orange juice every day. If it is challenging for you to consume these foods day in and day out, you may want to consider taking a vitamin D supplement daily.

Common Spices and Herbs That Ease Inflammation

Currently, there are many supplements and spices on the market that claim they can reduce inflammation and its associated pain in a natural manner, without side effects. Unfortunately, clinical research that supports these claims is sparse and most claims are solely anecdotal. Here are a few that have withstood the test of time:

- **Garlic** contains chemicals that crush inflammation-promoting substances. Regular garlic consumption can help minimize asthma symptoms and reduce the pain and inflammation caused by osteoarthritis and rheumatoid arthritis.
- **Curcumin** is a substance found in turmeric. It's touted as having antioxidant powers, anti-inflammatory qualities, and possibly even anticancer effects. Some researchers believe there is a link between higher curcumin intake and a lower incidence of Alzheimer's disease.
- **Ginger** is believed to inhibit biochemicals that promote inflammation, especially in cases of osteoarthritis and rheumatoid arthritis.

Hydrate for Health

Water is the most critical nutrient in our diets. Bodily fluids are necessary for digestion, absorption, and transportation of essential nutrients throughout the body. Adequate fluid intake can prevent headaches and fatigue, and enhance memory and circulation. Most importantly, studies have shown that individuals with rheumatoid arthritis fare better when properly hydrated, due to the cushioning and nurturing effect of water on the joints. The Institute of Medicine recommends that men consume 125 ounces of fluids and women consume 90 ounces of fluids every day.

After water, tea is the most commonly consumed beverage in the world. There are three main types of tea—green, oolong, and black. Green tea is made from unfermented leaves and contains the highest concentration of the potent antioxidants referred to as polyphenols. Oolong tea is prepared from partially fermented tea leaves, while black tea is fully fermented. Overall, the greater the degree of fermentation, the lower the polyphenol concentration and the higher the caffeine content, so green tea appears to be the most potent of the teas. The polyphenols, better known as catechins, found in green tea help neutralize free radicals and combat inflammation. In general, two to three cups of green tea per day are recommended to provide the therapeutic dose of 240 to 320 milligrams of polyphenols.

Move More

The anti-inflammatory effects of regular, moderate exercise help to lower the risk of heart disease, diabetes, high blood pressure, and osteoporosis. Active individuals possess lower levels of C-reactive protein (CRP), indicating less inflammation. The anti-inflammatory effect of exercise may be related to the increase in antioxidant production that occurs as a body becomes more fit. The extra internal antioxidants destroy free radicals associated with chronic inflammation.

> **fact**
>
> Individuals who exercise regularly are better equipped to deal with life's stressors and tend to experience a better sense of well-being, improved mood, and enhanced self-esteem.

Try to include aerobic exercise (walking, jogging, dancing, swimming) three times a week, weight training two times a week, and stretching after every workout.

Essential Sleep

Sleep is essential for your immune system to function optimally. Inadequate sleep can lead to an increased release of pro-inflammatory chemicals. A recent study found that sleep durations of six to eight hours were linked to significantly lower levels of the inflammatory markers in the blood compared to sleep durations of less than six hours. While you sleep, your body focuses on restoring and repairing. After a good night's sleep, the brain and body are more alert, and you are better able to concentrate and focus.

Try the following steps to encourage good sleep habits:

- Aim for seven to eight hours of sleep each night.
- Limit exposure to caffeine, large quantities of food, and stress within the two-hour period prior to sleep.
- Limit your screen time prior to sleep. Light-emitting devices can stimulate the brain and reduce the desire to snooze.
- Set a sleep schedule and keep with it as best you can both during weekdays and on weekends.
- Exercise each day in the morning or afternoon. Limit exercise as bedtime approaches to reduce the risk of getting a second wind.

The Stress-Cortisol-Inflammation Connection

Since the beginning of time, stress exposure has initiated a fight-or-flight response that causes an increased heart rate and body temperature, elevated blood pressure, and a rise in the stress hormone referred to as cortisol. This response results in the delivery of oxygen and nutrients to the parts of the body that need them most in hopes of allowing the body to successfully deal with the stress. Once the stressor is gone, blood pressure, heart rate, and other factors modified by the stress should return to normal.

You regularly experience "everyday" stressors related to your job, relationships, finances, overloaded schedule, and major life changes. Unfortunately, your body doesn't differentiate between "short-term" stressors and "chronic, everyday" stressors, so it continually secretes cortisol. Over time, chronic stress can result in consistently elevated blood pressure levels that can lead to nicks and injuries within the blood vessels. These microscopic tears eventually trigger an inflammatory response in the body as it attempts to mend the tears. Ultimately, this inflammation can lead to a heart attack or stroke.

Factors that increase cortisol levels include:

■ Caffeine consumption
■ Inadequate sleep
■ Severe trauma and stress
■ Intense or prolonged physical activity
■ Stressful commuting

However, there are some things that actually decrease cortisol levels:

■ Omega-3 fatty acids
■ Black tea
■ Yoga and other relaxation techniques
■ Massage therapy
■ Laughing

So, although some stress is good and can motivate you to achieve your short- and long-term goals, too much stress will ultimately lead to numerous health problems. For example, studies have found that individuals who are angry and hostile have higher CRP levels than people who are more laid-back. These elevated CRP levels indicate that inflammation is loitering in the body.

Unwind with Yoga

One recent study found that regularly practicing yoga can lower pro-inflammatory markers that rise as individuals age. Even after stressful experiences, the individuals who regularly practiced yoga showed smaller increases in inflammation in response to stress. Yoga helps you learn to manage everyday stressors more effectively. In a nutshell, yoga is a simple and enjoyable activity that can combat inflammation and subsequent disease.

Gentle Nutrition

While the role of nutrition in preventing inflammation and chronic disease has been clearly established by the scientific community, the importance of nutrition has created guilty eaters who feel the need to apologize for eating indulgent foods that may be considered "unhealthy." It's important to learn about the risk of chronic diseases, but the focus shouldn't be on the negatives, or on what *not* to eat, because dieting almost never works. Over 90 percent of people who start a new diet will regain all the weight they lost plus more shortly after the diet is over, and the cycle usually continues.

What if you took a different approach to encouraging health? Instead of focusing on scary statistics or the "bad" foods that may lead to chronic disease, we can focus on what we can add to our lives. Healthy eating is about eating a variety of foods and having a good relationship with food. You can help build the relationship by practicing gentle nutrition: feeding your body various foods—both nutritious and not as nutritious—and knowing that over the course of time, you're getting the nutrients you need. By gently respecting the needs of your body, you can add healthy foods that also taste delicious, all without dieting.

Diet and exercise alone are not the answers to a happy, healthy life. Focusing solely on these aspects takes the focus away from maintaining healthy relationships, self-care practices, positive self-talk, and attending to mental health. When you take care of yourself and treat your body with respect, health will come naturally.

CHAPTER 2

Breakfast

Coconut Turmeric Smoothie Bowls

SERVES 2

Per Serving

Calories	612
Fat	32g
Sodium	27mg
Carbohydrates	71g
Fiber	14g
Sugar	45g
Protein	10g

Indulge in the taste of the tropics without leaving home with these sunny smoothie bowls. The addition of turmeric adds anti-inflammatory power, while the fruit and nut toppings provide plenty of fiber, vitamins, and minerals.

½ cup orange juice

½ cup coconut milk

1 cup frozen pineapple chunks

1 cup frozen mango chunks

1 small banana, peeled and chopped

1 tablespoon ground flaxseed

¼ teaspoon ground turmeric

1 cup sliced strawberries

1 cup sliced kiwi

½ cup blueberries

½ cup chopped walnuts

½ cup unsweetened coconut flakes

1 Place orange juice, coconut milk, pineapple, mango, banana, flax-seed, and turmeric in a blender and process until smooth and creamy. Pour into two shallow bowls.

2 Top mixture with strawberries, kiwi, blueberries, walnuts, and coconut flakes and serve immediately.

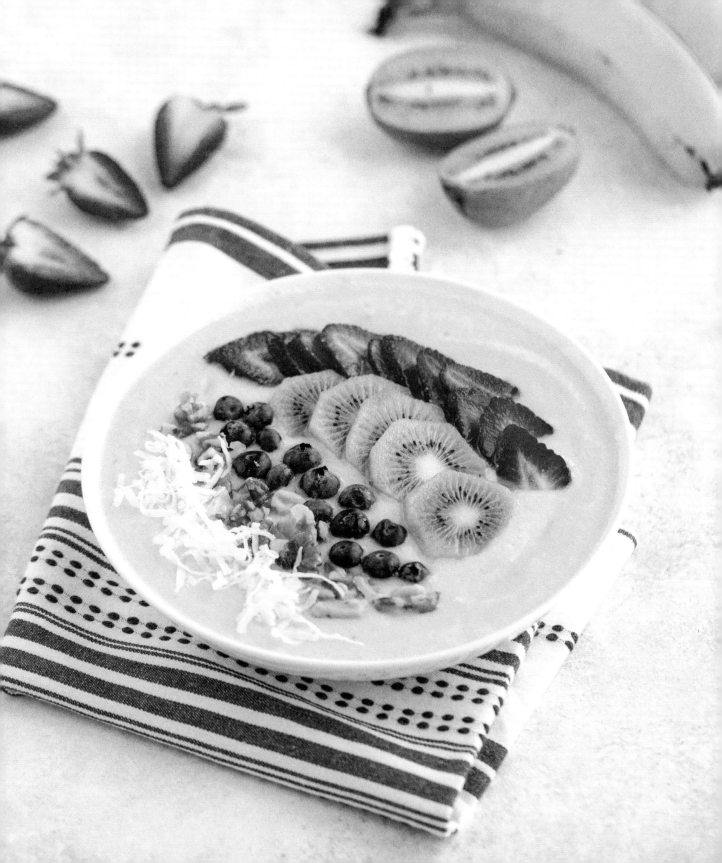

Strawberry Banana Smoothie

SERVES 2

Per Serving

Calories	212
Fat	3g
Sodium	62mg
Carbohydrates	45g
Fiber	3g
Sugar	31g
Protein	1g

BANANAS AND STRAWBERRIES

Bananas are a tasty source of soluble fiber. Strawberries have the added benefit of being high in both soluble and insoluble fiber in the form of pectin and seeds. Both bananas and strawberries are also higher in minerals than any other soft fruits.

A classic combination, strawberry and banana, forms the fiber-rich base of this breakfast treat. Try adding a scoop of vanilla protein powder to help you stay full longer.

1 medium banana, peeled and chopped

1 cup chopped frozen strawberries

1 cup low-fat vanilla frozen yogurt

¼ cup orange juice

1 teaspoon honey

Combine all ingredients in a blender and blend until smooth. Pour into two large glasses and serve immediately.

Peach Yogurt Smoothie

Greek yogurt adds thickness and protein to your morning smoothie. For a sorbet-like texture, use frozen peaches.

½ medium banana, peeled and chopped

1½ cups chopped peaches

1 cup low-fat vanilla Greek yogurt

¼ cup orange juice

1 teaspoon honey

Combine all ingredients in a blender and blend until smooth. Pour into two large glasses and serve immediately.

SERVES 2

Per Serving

Calories	228
Fat	3g
Sodium	47mg
Carbohydrates	37g
Fiber	3g
Sugar	30g
Protein	12g

FIBER FACT

If you use orange juice with pulp in it, you increase your fiber consumption without even thinking about it, so don't pick up the pulp-free variety any-more. The same goes for grapefruit juice.

Morning Sunshine Smoothie

SERVES 2

Per Serving

Calories	337
Fat	7g
Sodium	208mg
Carbohydrates	45g
Fiber	2g
Sugar	42g
Protein	24g

Pineapples are an unexpected source of flavonoids, an antioxidant that protects your body from chronic disease. Bromelain, an enzyme found in pineapples, may reduce the risk of cancer.

1 cup low-fat vanilla Greek yogurt

½ cup powdered skim milk

2 tablespoons flaxseed powder

2 tablespoons vanilla soy protein powder

2 tablespoons vanilla extract

1 cup chilled crushed pineapple

Combine all ingredients in a blender and blend until smooth. Pour into two large glasses and serve immediately.

Cornmeal Grits

SERVES 4

Per Serving

Calories	90
Fat	6g
Sodium	481mg
Carbohydrates	9g
Fiber	0g
Sugar	0g
Protein	0g

This warm cereal is similar to oatmeal. It can be eaten in a variety of ways: as a breakfast cereal, as a side with eggs, or with gravy. Try the grits with cheese stirred in and spicy sautéed shrimp on top.

4 cups water

1 teaspoon salt

1 cup polenta

2 tablespoons butter

1. Place water and salt in a medium saucepan and bring to a boil over high heat. Reduce heat to medium-low.
2. Gradually add polenta, stirring constantly, until thickened, about 15 minutes. Remove from heat and stir in butter.
3. Serve immediately for soft grits, or pour into a greased 9" × 5" loaf pan and let cool. When cool, grits can be sliced and fried or grilled.

Cinnamon Vanilla Nutty Granola

Serve this granola with fruit and yogurt or pack it into a small container for an on-the-go breakfast. Flaxseeds and sesame seeds are both rich in omega-3 fatty acids, which can help to lower blood pressure and cholesterol, and reduce joint pain and stiffness.

4 cups old-fashioned rolled oats

1 cup sliced almonds

½ teaspoon ground cinnamon

1 teaspoon vanilla extract

4 ounces orange blossom honey

2 tablespoons canola oil

½ cup wheat germ

¼ cup sesame seeds

¼ cup millet

¼ cup flaxseeds

1. Preheat oven to 350°F.
2. In a large bowl, toss together oats, almonds, cinnamon, vanilla, honey, and oil. Spread mixture on a large ungreased baking sheet and bake for 10 minutes.
3. Remove from oven and stir. Add wheat germ, sesame seeds, and millet and stir again. Bake for 15 minutes.
4. Remove from oven and stir. Add flaxseeds and stir again. Bake for 10 minutes.
5. Remove from oven and place pan on a wire rack to cool. Break up large chunks. Keep in a jar or covered container for up to 1 week.

SERVES 6

Per Serving

Calories	561
Fat	23g
Sodium	66mg
Carbohydrates	71g
Fiber	14g
Sugar	17g
Protein	18g

THE SCOOP ON MILLET

Millet is a whole grain that looks like tiny corn kernels and has a sweet, nutty flavor when toasted. Though technically a seed, it cooks like a whole grain such as rice or quinoa.

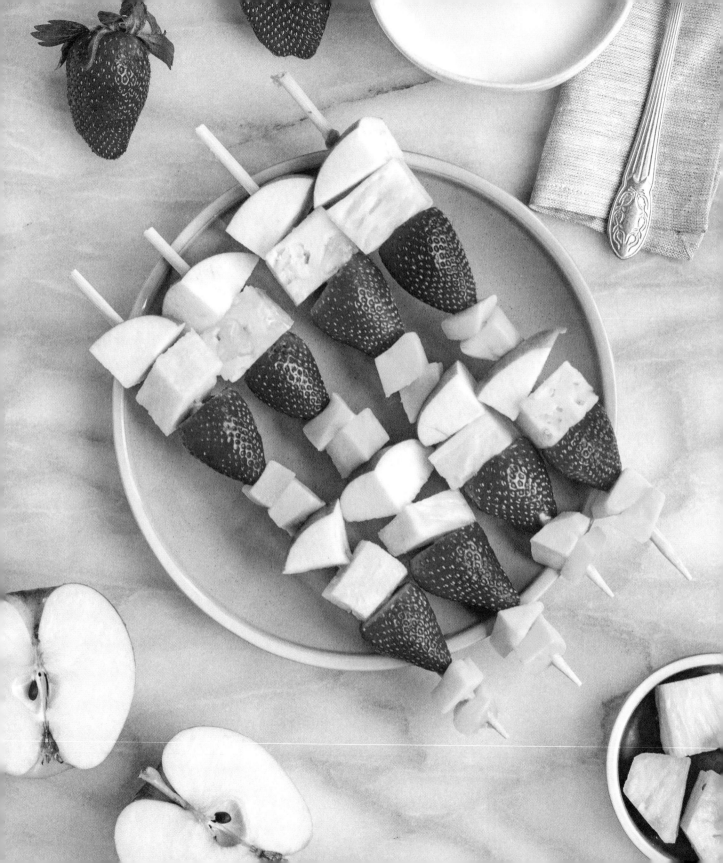

Fresh Fruit Kebabs with Vanilla Yogurt Sauce

Kebabs make a fun breakfast that's easy to prepare in advance. Choose fresh, ripe fruit for the best flavor and texture.

1 cup diced apple (1" cubes)

1 cup diced pineapple (1" cubes)

8 small strawberries, hulled

1 cup diced mango (1" cubes)

¾ cup whole-milk vanilla yogurt

¼ cup heavy cream

½ teaspoon vanilla extract

SERVES 4

Per Serving

Calories	162
Fat	7g
Sodium	31mg
Carbohydrates	22g
Fiber	2g
Sugar	13g
Protein	4g

1 Alternately thread apple cubes, pineapple cubes, strawberries, and mango cubes onto four wooden skewers. Repeat until all the fruit is used.

2 Whisk together yogurt, cream, and vanilla in a small bowl. Serve kebabs with dipping sauce on the side.

Crepes with Blueberry Sauce

For a savory dish, omit the blueberry sauce and wrap the crepes around roasted vegetables and Walnut Parsley Pesto (see recipe in Chapter 6).

SERVES 8

Per Serving

Calories	197
Fat	7g
Sodium	229mg
Carbohydrates	27g
Fiber	4g
Sugar	11g
Protein	7g

HERBAL SWEETENER

Stevia is an herbal sugar-free sweetener, and it can help balance blood sugar levels. It is three hundred times sweeter than regular sugar and is heat-stable. Finally, a great alternative to refined and artificial sweeteners!

4 large eggs

1 cup soy or rice milk

1½ cups water, divided

½ teaspoon salt

1 cup spelt flour

3 tablespoons melted butter

1 medium apple, peeled, cored, and thinly sliced

1 medium pear, peeled, cored, and thinly sliced

2 cups blueberries

1 teaspoon stevia powder

1 tablespoon cornstarch

1 teaspoon ground cinnamon

1 Combine eggs, soy milk, ½ cup water, salt, flour, and butter in a blender; purée until smooth. Refrigerate for at least 2 hours or overnight.

2 Heat a 10" crepe pan over medium heat and spray with nonstick cooking spray. When pan is hot, pour ¼ cup batter onto pan and swirl around to cover the bottom. Cook until browned on bottom, about 1 minute.

3 Loosen the crepe with a spatula, then flip carefully. Cook the second side for 30 seconds. Stack crepes on a plate and cover with a cloth towel until all the batter is used.

4 Place apple, pear, blueberries, stevia, and ½ cup water in a medium heavy saucepan over medium heat. Cook, stirring occasionally, until mixture just comes to a boil. Reduce heat to medium-low and simmer until fruit is tender, about 10 minutes.

5 Dissolve cornstarch in remaining ½ cup water. Stir cornstarch mixture into fruit mixture and stir until thickened, about 30 seconds. Remove from heat and set aside. Keep warm.

6 Lay out a crepe on a plate and spoon some of the fruit mixture onto one half of the crepe. Fold the crepe over and sprinkle with some of the cinnamon. Repeat with remaining crepes, sauce, and cinnamon. Serve immediately.

Banana–Oat Bran Waffles

Use either a nonstick standard waffle iron or a nonstick Belgian waffle maker—choose the latter for waffles with deep indentations to hold pools of maple syrup. Bananas are a good source of vitamin C and an excellent source of vitamin B_6, both essential to maintaining a healthy immune system.

2 large eggs or ½ cup egg substitute

1 cup buttermilk

2 very ripe medium bananas, peeled and chopped

4 tablespoons melted butter

½ cup all-purpose flour

½ cup 100% whole-wheat flour

½ cup oat bran

2 teaspoons baking powder

½ teaspoon salt

½ cup finely chopped pecans

1   Preheat a waffle iron and spray both surfaces with nonstick cooking spray.

2   In a large bowl, beat together eggs, buttermilk, bananas, and butter until well blended and smooth, about 1 minute. Fold in flours, oat bran, baking powder, and salt, stirring until just combined and moistened; the batter should be stiff, not runny. Fold in pecans.

3   Cook waffles according to the manufacturer's directions. Serve hot.

SERVES 4

Per Serving

Calories	457
Fat	24g
Sodium	391mg
Carbohydrates	49g
Fiber	7g
Sugar	10g
Protein	13g

WHY OAT BRAN?

Because it is so high in fiber, oat bran is often touted as one of the soluble-fiber foods that helps lower cholesterol levels in the blood. It also adds texture and a delicate nutty flavor to a wide range of dishes, including cereals, baked goods, soups, and stews.

Blackberry Buckwheat Pancakes

SERVES 4

Per Serving

Calories	405
Fat	15g
Sodium	390mg
Carbohydrates	56g
Fiber	3g
Sugar	15g
Protein	13g

THE FRUIT OF KNOWLEDGE

Although many people believe that buckwheat is a cereal grain, it is actually a fruit. It's ideal for people who are sensitive to wheat or other grains that contain protein glutens. Not only is this fruit used in gluten-free foods, but you'll also find it added to energy bars and meatless entrées.

The seeds of blackberries are a good source of fiber, omega-3 fatty acids, and protein. Best of all, fresh or frozen blackberries are available to enjoy year-round.

½ cup all-purpose flour

½ cup 100% whole-wheat flour

½ cup buckwheat flour

3 tablespoons sugar

1½ teaspoons baking powder

1 teaspoon baking soda

½ teaspoon salt

2 large eggs or ½ cup egg substitute

3 tablespoons melted butter

1½ cups buttermilk

2 teaspoons vegetable oil, divided

1 cup blackberries

1 In a large bowl, whisk together flours, sugar, baking powder, baking soda, and salt.

2 In a medium bowl, whisk together eggs, butter, and buttermilk.

3 Stir egg mixture into flour mixture until just combined. There will be lumps; be careful not to overmix.

4 Brush a griddle or large skillet with 1 teaspoon oil and place over medium heat. Pour about ⅓ cup batter for each pancake onto hot griddle or pan. Scatter several blackberries on top of batter. Flip pancake when bubbles have formed and started to pop through the batter, about 2 minutes. Cook on other side for 1 minute. Repeat with remaining batter and blackberries, adding remaining oil to the pan when necessary.

5 Serve hot.

"Sausage" Bread Pudding

Vary the berry topping to suit your taste by using raspberries, blueberries, blackberries, or strawberries. Or substitute 2 cups of your favorite seasonal fruits cut into small pieces.

1 tablespoon olive oil

1 teaspoon minced garlic

1 cup crumbled soy "sausage" meat

1 teaspoon Cajun or Creole seasoning

2 cups low-fat milk

3 tablespoons melted butter

4 large eggs or 1 cup egg substitute

2 cups shredded low-fat Cheddar or Monterey jack cheese

3 cups cubed sourdough bread

2 cups fresh blackberries or blueberries

1 Preheat oven to 375°F. Lightly butter a 2-quart baking dish.

2 Heat oil in a large skillet over medium heat and sauté garlic for 30 seconds. Add soy "sausage" to the skillet and sprinkle with Cajun seasoning. Cook, stirring occasionally, for 5 minutes or until soy "sausage" is hot. Remove from heat.

3 In a large bowl, beat together milk, butter, and eggs until foamy, about 1 minute. Stir in cheese and "sausage" mixture. Place bread in the prepared baking dish and pour milk mixture over bread.

4 Bake for 45 minutes or until puffy and golden. Top pudding with berries and serve hot.

SERVES 4

Per Serving

Calories	566
Fat	32g
Sodium	871mg
Carbohydrates	36g
Fiber	6g
Sugar	11g
Protein	30g

WHAT ARE SOY "SAUSAGES"?

Made from soy proteins, soy "sausages" are available as links or as a compact product packed in a tube. In the tube, the soy meat is easy to crumble and sauté like its pork sausage counterpart; alternatively, it slices easily and pan-fries like a patty. Look for soy "sausage" products in a refrigerated case displayed with other vegetarian and vegan items.

Cheezy Tofu, Potato, and Pepper Breakfast Casserole

SERVES 6

Per Serving

Calories	188
Fat	11g
Sodium	233mg
Carbohydrates	15g
Fiber	3g
Sugar	1g
Protein	8g

Here's the perfect brunch casserole—it's delicious, satisfying, and loaded with plant-based protein.

1 tablespoon plant-based butter

1 (14-ounce) block extra-firm tofu, drained and pressed

½ teaspoon garlic powder

½ teaspoon onion powder

¼ teaspoon salt

¼ teaspoon ground turmeric

3 tablespoons vegetable broth

1 tablespoon avocado oil

1 (16-ounce) bag frozen hash brown potatoes

1 medium red bell pepper, seeded and diced

½ cup sliced scallions

½ cup shredded vegan Cheddar cheese

1 Preheat oven to 425°F.

2 Melt butter in a large skillet over medium heat. Crumble in tofu and add garlic powder, onion powder, salt, and turmeric. Stir in broth. Transfer mixture to a large bowl.

3 Wipe out skillet with paper towels. Return to medium heat and add oil. Add potatoes and bell pepper and sauté until the potatoes are crisp and brown, 10–15 minutes. Stir in scallions and vegan cheese, then add potato mixture to tofu mixture. Stir to combine.

4 Spread mixture into an ungreased 9" × 13" baking dish. Bake for 20 minutes.

5 Set aside to cool for 5 minutes before serving.

Edamame Omelet

The addition of cheese turns this into a fusion dish. To add more Asian flavor, omit the cheese and stir in some shredded daikon and crushed chilies.

3 tablespoons olive oil, divided

1 teaspoon minced garlic

1 bunch scallions, trimmed and cut into 1" pieces

½ cup shelled edamame

1 tablespoon low-sodium soy sauce

3 large eggs or ¾ cup egg substitute, beaten

½ cup shredded Cheddar cheese

1 tablespoon chopped fresh cilantro

SERVES 2	
Per Serving	
Calories	381
Fat	34g
Sodium	541mg
Carbohydrates	5g
Fiber	1g
Sugar	1g
Protein	12g

1 Heat 2 tablespoons oil in a small skillet over medium heat and sauté garlic and scallions for 2 minutes. Add edamame and soy sauce and sauté 1 minute more. Remove edamame mixture from the skillet and set aside.

2 Heat remaining 1 tablespoon oil in the same skillet over medium heat. Pour in eggs and scatter cheese on top. Lift up the edges of the omelet, tipping the skillet back and forth to cook eggs for 1–2 minutes until the top appears firm. Sprinkle scallion mixture over one half of omelet and fold the other half over top.

3 Carefully lift omelet out of the skillet. Divide it in half, sprinkle with cilantro, and serve.

Vegan Eggs Benedict with Smoky Tempeh Bacon

SERVES 4

Per Serving

Calories	491
Fat	24g
Sodium	784mg
Carbohydrates	39g
Fiber	10g
Sugar	6g
Protein	29g

It takes a little extra time to make eggs Benedict, but it's totally worth it for a lazy weekend breakfast. Tempeh is a plant-based protein source made from fermented soybeans. Combined with liquid smoke and spices, it tastes very similar to bacon!

2 tablespoons liquid smoke

2 tablespoons soy sauce

1 teaspoon barbecue sauce

¼ teaspoon smoked paprika

1 (8-ounce) package tempeh, thinly sliced

1 cup vegetable broth

1 cup raw cashews

¼ cup nutritional yeast

2 tablespoons lemon juice

1 teaspoon apple cider vinegar

½ teaspoon ground turmeric

1 tablespoon vegan Dijon mustard

1 teaspoon garlic powder

1 teaspoon onion powder

1 cup Just Egg vegan egg replacement

4 whole-wheat vegan English muffins, split and toasted

1 medium tomato, sliced

2 tablespoons balsamic glaze

1 medium avocado, peeled, pitted, and sliced

1 Preheat oven to 350° F. Line a large baking sheet with parchment paper.

2 In a large bowl, whisk together liquid smoke, soy sauce, barbecue sauce, and paprika. Add tempeh slices and turn to coat. Set aside to marinate at room temperature for 15 minutes.

3 Use tongs to remove tempeh slices from marinade and place them on the prepared baking sheet. Discard any remaining marinade. Bake for 10 minutes, flip, and bake for another 10 minutes or until crispy. Remove from oven and set aside to cool.

4 In a small saucepan over high heat, bring broth to a boil. Place cashews in a small heatproof bowl. Pour hot broth over cashews and set aside for 15 minutes. Then pour cashews and broth into a blender. Add nutritional yeast, lemon juice, vinegar, turmeric, mustard, garlic powder, and onion powder. Blend until smooth. Add ¼ to ½ cup warm water if needed to create a smooth, creamy consistency. Transfer sauce to a small saucepan and heat over low heat until warmed through.

5 Heat a medium nonstick skillet over medium heat. Add egg replacement and cook, stirring occasionally, for 4–5 minutes until set.

6 On each of four small plates, place 2 English muffin halves. Top with egg replacement, tempeh, tomato, balsamic glaze, and avocado slices. Pour cashew mixture over the muffins. Serve immediately.

Spinach, Mushroom, and Tomato Tofu Scramble

SERVES 4

Per Serving

Calories	246
Fat	12g
Sodium	637mg
Carbohydrates	16g
Fiber	6g
Sugar	6g
Protein	18g

When tofu is scrambled with oil and spices, it transforms into an egg-like texture. Turmeric provides the yellow color and a healthy dose of antioxidant power.

2 tablespoons extra-virgin olive oil

1 medium yellow onion, peeled and diced

3 cloves garlic, peeled and minced

8 ounces cremini mushrooms, thinly sliced

1 (14-ounce) package extra-firm tofu, drained and pressed

1 pint grape tomatoes, halved

1 teaspoon ground turmeric

1 teaspoon salt

½ teaspoon dried basil

½ teaspoon dried oregano

5 ounces baby spinach, roughly chopped

1 Heat oil in a large skillet over medium heat. Sauté onion until softened, 3–4 minutes. Add garlic and sauté for 30 seconds.

2 Add mushrooms in a single layer. Let cook undisturbed for about 5 minutes until they begin to brown on one side. Flip and cook for another 5 minutes or until mushrooms are golden brown.

3 Crumble tofu into the skillet and stir to combine. Add tomatoes, turmeric, salt, basil, and oregano. Cook, stirring occasionally, for 5 minutes.

4 Add spinach to the skillet and stir until wilted, about 2 minutes. Serve hot.

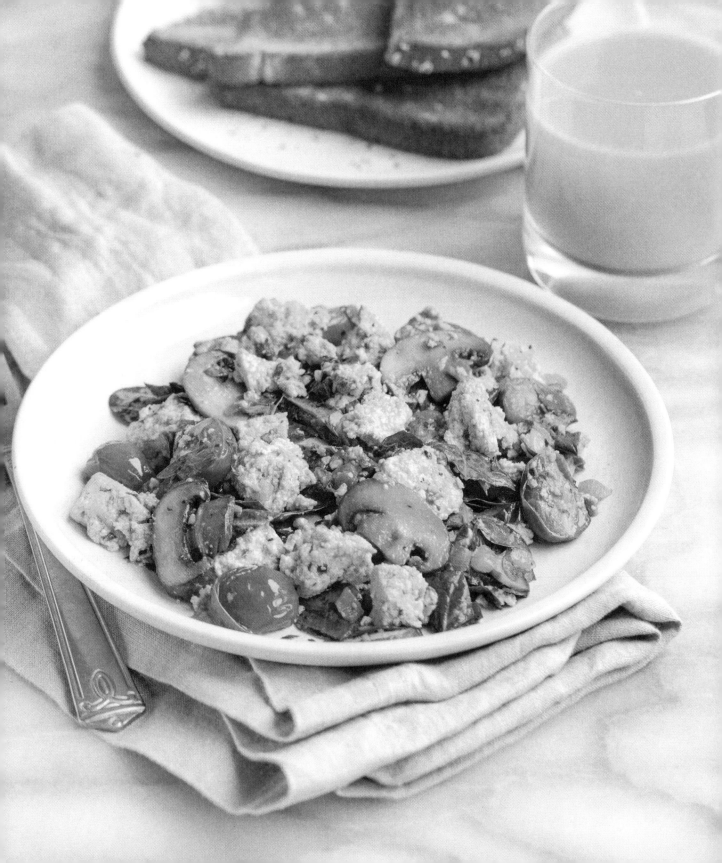

Savory Steel-Cut Oatmeal with Avocado and Fried Eggs

Per Serving

Calories	637
Fat	35g
Sodium	768mg
Carbohydrates	41g
Fiber	6g
Sugar	6g
Protein	41g

STEEL-CUT POWER

Steel-cut oats are slightly higher in fiber than old-fashioned or quick oats. They are also a prebiotic food, which means they promote the growth of beneficial intestinal bacteria.

Steel-cut oatmeal can be prepared in large batches for weekly meal prep and stored in the refrigerator. Oats can be reheated in the microwave or on the stove. Add a splash of milk if the mixture seems too thick.

2 teaspoons extra-virgin olive oil, divided

¼ cup steel-cut oats

1 cup water

½ cup low-fat cottage cheese

2 tablespoons grated Parmesan cheese

⅛ teaspoon salt

⅛ teaspoon ground black pepper

½ teaspoon sriracha

2 large eggs

½ small avocado, peeled, pitted, and sliced

1 Heat 1 teaspoon oil in a small saucepan over medium heat. Add oats and stir to toast for 2–3 minutes until fragrant. Add water, increase heat to high, and bring to a boil. Reduce heat to low, cover, and simmer for 20 minutes, stirring occasionally.

2 Remove pan from heat and stir in cottage cheese, Parmesan cheese, salt, pepper, and sriracha. Set aside and keep warm.

3 Heat remaining 1 teaspoon oil in a small skillet over medium heat. Gently crack eggs into the skillet and cook until the whites are almost solid, about 3 minutes, then flip and cook for 20 seconds.

4 Pour oats into a wide, shallow bowl and top with avocado and fried eggs. Serve immediately.

Apple Bread

Moist and full of apples, this bread is great for breakfast or as a snack with a piece of Cheddar cheese. The whole-wheat flour and apples provide a healthy dose of fiber.

1 (0.25-ounce) packet yeast

4 tablespoons sugar, divided

1⅓ cups warm water, divided

3 tablespoons butter, softened

1 teaspoon salt

¼ teaspoon baking powder

1¾ cups all-purpose flour

1¾ cups whole-wheat flour

1 tablespoon vegetable oil

1 teaspoon ground cinnamon

1 cup peeled, chopped apples

SERVES 8

Per Serving

Calories	288
Fat	7g
Sodium	326mg
Carbohydrates	49g
Fiber	5g
Sugar	10g
Protein	7g

1. Combine yeast, 1 teaspoon sugar, and ⅓ cup water in a small bowl. Let sit for 5 minutes.

2. To the bowl of a stand mixer, add remaining 1 cup water, 2⅔ tablespoons sugar, butter, salt, and baking powder and mix until combined. Mix in all-purpose flour and then the yeast mixture. Add whole-wheat flour and knead with a dough hook attachment for 10 minutes.

3. Brush oil on the inside of a large bowl. Place dough in bowl and turn to coat with oil. Cover and let rise in a warm place for 1–2 hours until doubled in bulk.

4. Oil a 9" × 5" loaf pan. In a small bowl, combine cinnamon with remaining 1 tablespoon sugar. Set aside.

5. Punch down dough, then roll it into a 9" × 12" rectangle on a floured work surface. Scatter apples over the dough and sprinkle with cinnamon and sugar mixture. Starting with one short side, roll dough into a cylinder and place in the prepared pan. Cover and let it rise in a warm place for 90 minutes or until doubled in size.

6. Preheat oven to 350°F.

7. Uncover dough and bake for 50 minutes. Cool in pan for 10 minutes, then transfer to a wire rack to cool completely.

100% WHOLE-WHEAT TAKEOVER

If you want to boost the nutritional payoff of your recipes, you can replace white (all-purpose) flour with whole-wheat flour by substituting one for one. However, products made with whole-wheat flour will be denser. Try sifting the flour a few extra times to incorporate more air, which will result in a lighter, more tender final product.

Cinnamon Swirl Raisin Bread

SERVES 8	
Per Serving	
Calories	327
Fat	5g
Sodium	321mg
Carbohydrates	60g
Fiber	5g
Sugar	19g
Protein	7g

Toast this bread for a delicious and filling start to a long day. The whole-wheat flour provides fiber, while the raisins add some iron and vitamin B_6, which supports a healthy immune system.

1 (0.25-ounce) packet yeast
3 tablespoons sugar, divided
1⅓ cups warm water, divided
3 tablespoons butter, softened
1 teaspoon salt
¼ teaspoon baking powder
1¾ cups all-purpose flour
1¾ cups whole-wheat flour
1 cup raisins
1 tablespoon vegetable oil
3 tablespoons ground cinnamon

1. Combine yeast, 1 teaspoon sugar, and ⅓ cup water in a small bowl. Let sit for 5 minutes.
2. To the bowl of a stand mixer, add remaining 1 cup water and 2⅔ tablespoons sugar, butter, salt, and baking powder and mix until combined. Mix in all-purpose flour and then the yeast mixture. Add whole-wheat flour and raisins and knead with a dough hook for 10 minutes.
3. Brush oil on the inside of a large bowl. Place dough in bowl and turn to coat with oil. Cover and let rise in a warm place for 1–2 hours until doubled in bulk.
4. Oil a 9" × 5" loaf pan.
5. Punch down dough, then roll it into a 9" × 12" rectangle on a floured work surface. Sprinkle with cinnamon. Starting with one short side, roll dough into a cylinder and place in the prepared pan. Cover and let it rise in a warm place for 90 minutes or until doubled in size.
6. Preheat oven to 350°F.
7. Uncover dough and bake for 40 minutes. Cool in pan for 10 minutes, then transfer to a wire rack to cool completely.

Raisin Bran Muffins

A breakfast of a glass of orange juice (with pulp) and a bran muffin is a delicious way to start your day with fiber. Substitute half of the all-purpose flour with whole-wheat flour to add even more fiber.

1 cup boiling water

2½ cups All-Bran cereal, divided

2½ cups all-purpose flour

2½ teaspoons baking soda

1 teaspoon salt

½ cup vegetable oil

1 cup sugar

2 large eggs, beaten

2 cups buttermilk

1½ cups raisins

1 cup bran flakes

1 Preheat oven to 400°F. Grease three twelve-cup muffin tins or line them with paper cups.

2 Pour boiling water over 1 cup All-Bran cereal in a large bowl and set aside for 10 minutes.

3 In a medium bowl, stir together flour, baking soda, and salt. Set aside.

4 Add oil to the bran and water mixture and stir to combine. Stir in remaining 1½ cups All-Bran cereal, sugar, eggs, and buttermilk.

5 Add the flour mixture to the bran mixture and stir to combine. Stir in raisins and bran flakes.

6 Fill muffin cups ¾ full with the batter and bake for 20 minutes. Cool muffins in muffin tins for 5 minutes, then transfer to a wire rack.

MAKES 36 MUFFINS

Per Serving (1 muffin)

Calories	121
Fat	4g
Sodium	102mg
Carbohydrates	20g
Fiber	1g
Sugar	11g
Protein	2g

QUICK BREADS VERSUS MUFFINS

Most quick-bread recipes can be used for muffins. You will get a dozen standard muffins or twenty-four mini-muffins. Always prepare your muffin tins with nonstick spray, even those tins that are supposedly nonstick. Muffins bake in about 15–20 minutes and make nice equal portions. Never overfill the muffin cups or the dough will rise and lap over the pan.

Blueberry Almond Breakfast Bars

SERVES 6

Per Serving

Calories	558
Fat	22g
Sodium	438mg
Carbohydrates	79g
Fiber	7g
Sugar	23g
Protein	10g

Deliciously portable, these nutrient-packed goodies taste like a cross between a granola bar and a blueberry muffin. Antioxidant blueberries have been linked to a reduced risk of cognitive decline and can improve short-term memory and motor coordination.

½ cup butter, softened

¾ cup firmly packed dark brown sugar

½ cup granulated sugar

2 large eggs or ½ cup egg substitute

1 teaspoon vanilla extract

2 cups old-fashioned rolled oats

1 cup 100% whole-wheat flour

1 teaspoon baking powder

1 teaspoon salt

2 cups blueberries

½ cup slivered almonds

1. Preheat oven to 350°F. Butter and flour an 8" × 8" baking pan.
2. In the bowl of a stand mixer, beat butter with brown sugar and granulated sugar until creamy, about 1 minute. Add eggs, one at a time, beating well after each addition. Beat in vanilla.
3. Stir or beat in oats, flour, baking powder, and salt until well combined. Fold in blueberries and almonds. Spoon mixture into the prepared pan.
4. Bake for 40 minutes or until the center feels firm, the edges are brown, and a toothpick inserted in the center comes out clean. Cool in pan for at least 1 hour. Slice into squares and serve.

CHAPTER 3

Appetizers and Snacks

Creamy Spinach Artichoke Dip

SERVES 6

Per Serving

Calories	173
Fat	10g
Sodium	479mg
Carbohydrates	13g
Fiber	3g
Sugar	3g
Protein	8g

This vegan version of a party favorite can be served with fresh vegetables, like baby carrots, celery sticks, lightly steamed broccoli florets, and bell pepper strips. It's also good with whole-grain crackers or pita triangles.

1 cup raw cashews

2 cups vegetable broth

½ cup nutritional yeast

2 tablespoons arrowroot starch

1 tablespoon apple cider vinegar

1 teaspoon salt

1 tablespoon olive oil

1 medium yellow onion, peeled and diced

2 cloves garlic, peeled and minced

5 ounces baby spinach, roughly chopped

1 (15-ounce) can water- or brine-packed artichoke hearts (not marinated), drained and chopped

1 Place cashews in a medium heatproof bowl. In a small saucepan over high heat, bring broth to a boil. Remove pan from heat and pour broth over cashews. Set aside for 15 minutes.

2 Transfer cashew mixture to a blender. Add nutritional yeast, arrowroot starch, vinegar, and salt and purée until smooth.

3 Preheat broiler to high. Place a rack in the upper third of the oven.

4 Heat oil in a large skillet over medium heat. Sauté onion until softened, 3–4 minutes. Add garlic and sauté for 30 seconds. Stir in puréed cashew mixture.

5 Add spinach and artichokes to the skillet and cook, stirring often, until thickened, 5–6 minutes.

6 Transfer mixture to a medium ungreased baking pan. Broil for 3–5 minutes until browned and set. Serve hot.

Fresh Pepper Salsa

Bell peppers are excellent sources of the antioxidant vitamins A and C. Chili peppers also contain capsaicin, which is a powerful anti-inflammatory compound.

1 medium yellow bell pepper, seeded and quartered

1 medium orange bell pepper, seeded and quartered

2 small jalapeño peppers, stemmed

2 small poblano chilies, stemmed

2 medium Anaheim chilies, stemmed

2 cloves garlic, peeled

¼ medium red onion, peeled

1 tablespoon lime juice

2 tablespoons canola oil

½ teaspoon cracked black pepper

¼ cup chopped fresh cilantro

1 Place bell peppers, jalapeño peppers, chilies, garlic, onion, and lime juice in a food processor and pulse until desired chunkiness is reached.

2 In a medium saucepan, heat oil over high heat until slightly smoking. Add pepper mixture and season with black pepper. Cook for 10 minutes, stirring occasionally.

3 Remove from heat and sprinkle with cilantro. Serve hot, cold, or at room temperature.

MAKES 1 PINT

Per Serving (¼ cup)

Calories	77
Fat	5g
Sodium	33mg
Carbohydrates	6g
Fiber	2g
Sugar	1g
Protein	2g

Vegan Queso

SERVES 8

Per Serving

Calories	314
Fat	18g
Sodium	681mg
Carbohydrates	25g
Fiber	4g
Sugar	7g
Protein	13g

Raw cashews have a wonderful creamy texture that can thicken many vegan dishes. Once soaked in boiling water for at least 15 minutes, they can be blended into a smooth cashew cream.

¾ cup raw cashews

1 cup vegetable broth

2 medium Yukon Gold potatoes, peeled and diced

4 cloves garlic, peeled

1½ tablespoons lemon juice

1 cup full-fat coconut milk

1 tablespoon nutritional yeast

1 teaspoon ground cumin

½ teaspoon smoked paprika

2 teaspoons salt

1 tablespoon extra-virgin olive oil

1 pound vegan crumbles (ground meat substitute)

1 (1-ounce) packet taco seasoning

1 (4-ounce) can pickled jalapeños, drained (reserve liquid)

1 (4-ounce) can green chilies, drained

1 (14.5-ounce) can petite-diced tomatoes

½ cup chopped fresh cilantro

1 Place cashews in a medium heatproof bowl. In a small saucepan over high heat, bring broth to a boil. Remove pan from heat and pour broth over cashews. Set aside for 15 minutes.

2 Place potatoes in a medium saucepan and cover with hot water. Bring to a boil over high heat, then cover and reduce heat to low. Simmer for about 10 minutes or until potatoes are fork-tender. Drain and transfer to a blender.

3 Add garlic, lemon juice, coconut milk, nutritional yeast, cumin, paprika, salt, and cashew mixture to the blender. Purée until smooth. Transfer to a large saucepan and set aside.

4 Heat oil in a large skillet over medium heat. Add vegan crumbles and sauté until browned, about 10 minutes. Stir in taco seasoning and the jalapeño liquid, then transfer to the large saucepan. Stir to combine.

5 Add jalapeños, green chilies, and tomatoes. Cook over low heat, stirring occasionally, until heated through, about 5 minutes.

6 Top with cilantro before serving.

Groovy Guacamole

Avocados may be high in fat, but they contain the good anti-inflammatory, monounsaturated type. Avocados are also favorably high in fiber, potassium, many B vitamins, and vitamin E.

2 large ripe avocados, peeled, pitted, and coarsely chopped

1 small white onion, peeled and diced

1 medium tomato, unpeeled and diced

1 small jalapeño pepper, stemmed and thinly sliced

2 tablespoons lime juice

½ teaspoon salt

Gently combine all ingredients in a serving bowl. Serve immediately or refrigerate, covered, for up to 1 day.

SERVES 4	
Per Serving	
Calories	201
Fat	16g
Sodium	302mg
Carbohydrates	12g
Fiber	8g
Sugar	3g
Protein	2g

AVOCADOS 101

Avocados darken easily when exposed to air, so it is best to save any leftovers with the pits and keep them in a tightly sealed container in the refrigerator. The use of lemon and lime juice in recipes will also keep discoloration at bay.

Traditional Hummus

Hummus is a popular dish throughout the Middle East and Mediterranean regions. It's a great source of iron and vitamin C, making it ideal for vegetarians and vegans. It also offers plenty of protein, fiber, and heart-healthy fats.

SERVES 6

Per Serving

Calories	94
Fat	6g
Sodium	363mg
Carbohydrates	8g
Fiber	2g
Sugar	1g
Protein	2g

HUMMUS MIX-INS

To make hummus a little more interesting, try adding a few slices of roasted red bell peppers to the food processor. Or top finished hummus with pico de gallo.

1 cup cooked chickpeas

½ bulb roasted garlic, peeled and chopped (1½ teaspoons)

2 tablespoons tahini

1 tablespoon grated lemon zest

3 tablespoons lemon juice

2 teaspoons extra-virgin olive oil

¾ teaspoon salt

½ teaspoon cracked black pepper

¼ cup chopped fresh parsley

1 Purée chickpeas in a blender or food processor. Add garlic, tahini, lemon zest, and juice. Continue to purée until mixture is thoroughly combined.

2 While continuing to purée, drizzle in oil in a stream until oil is incorporated and the mixture is smooth.

3 Transfer mixture to a small serving bowl. Season with salt and pepper and sprinkle with parsley before serving.

Sicilian Eggplant Caponata

Caponata is a traditional Italian dish made of eggplant sautéed in olive oil, tomato sauce, olives, capers, and an irresistible sweet and sour sauce.

1 large eggplant

2 tablespoons extra-virgin olive oil

½ small yellow onion, peeled and diced

2 stalks celery, trimmed and diced

1 medium red bell pepper, seeded and diced

2 cloves garlic, peeled and minced

1 (15-ounce) can crushed tomatoes

1 teaspoon salt

1 tablespoon capers

2 tablespoons minced green olives

2 tablespoons sugar

2 tablespoons white wine vinegar

1 (8-ounce) French-style baguette, thinly sliced

½ cup grated Parmesan cheese

SERVES 6	
Per Serving	
Calories	243
Fat	8g
Sodium	672mg
Carbohydrates	36g
Fiber	5g
Sugar	11g
Protein	7g

1 Preheat oven to 450°F.

2 Cut eggplant in half lengthwise and use a sharp knife to score several vertical cuts down the middle (don't cut all the way through). Place flesh side down on an ungreased baking sheet and roast for 15 minutes. Remove from oven and set aside to cool for 5 minutes. Scoop out eggplant from the skin and dice into small pieces. Set aside.

3 Heat oil in a large skillet over medium heat. Sauté onion, celery, and bell pepper for 5–7 minutes until tender. Add garlic and sauté 30 seconds.

4 Stir in eggplant, tomatoes, and salt. Cook over medium-low heat for about 10 minutes, stirring occasionally, until slightly thickened.

5 Add capers, olives, sugar, and vinegar to the skillet. Reduce heat to low and simmer for about 30 minutes, stirring often, until the mixture is very thick. Remove from heat and allow to cool to room temperature.

6 To serve, spread eggplant mixture on baguette slices and sprinkle with Parmesan cheese.

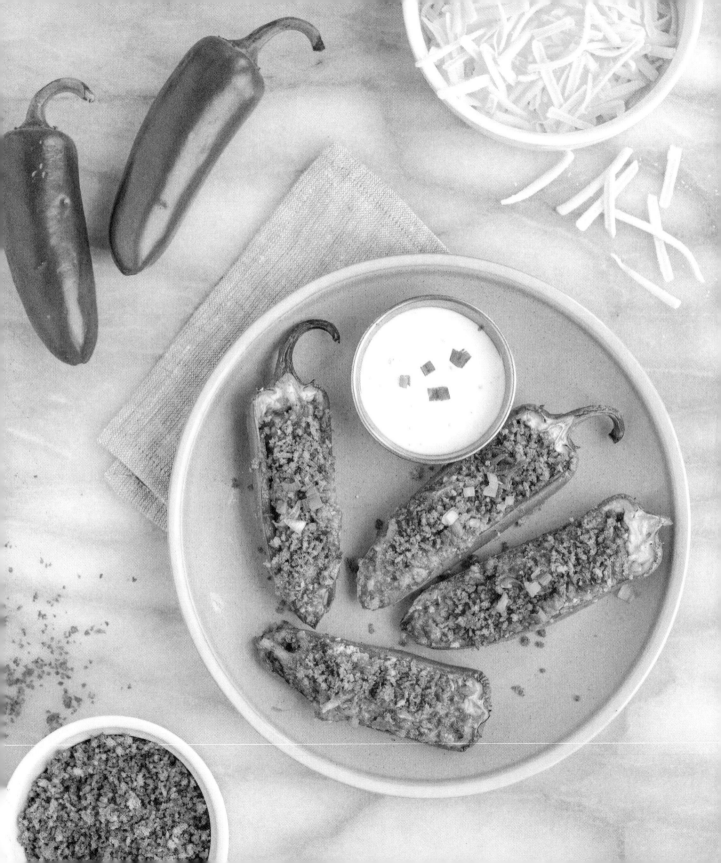

Vegan Sausage–Stuffed Jalapeño Poppers

Stuffed jalapeños are a crowd-pleasing game-day classic. Here's a plant-based version using vegan cheeses and sausage substitute.

12 medium jalapeño peppers

2 (14-ounce) Impossible Foods Plant Based Savory Sausage Chubs

1 cup shredded vegan Cheddar cheese

8 ounces vegan cream cheese, softened

½ tablespoon soy sauce

½ cup panko bread crumbs

1 Preheat oven to 400° F. Line two baking sheets with parchment paper.

2 Slice jalapeños in half lengthwise. Use a small spoon to scoop out the seeds.

3 In a large bowl, combine vegan sausage, vegan cheeses, and soy sauce. Scoop a rounded tablespoon of the mixture into each jalapeño half and place on the prepared baking sheets. Bake for 15 minutes.

4 Remove baking sheets from oven and top jalapeños with panko, then bake for 10 minutes more or until crispy.

5 Serve warm.

SERVES 6

Per Serving

Calories	568
Fat	37g
Sodium	1,012mg
Carbohydrates	35g
Fiber	4g
Sugar	1g
Protein	23g

PLANT-BASED MEAT SUBSTITUTES

There are many new plant-based meat substitutes on the market that not only taste delicious, but also look almost like the real thing. You can use them in dishes like meatloaf, or you can brown them to use in tacos or meat sauces. The key to getting nicely browned faux meat is to let it sit undisturbed until a nice crust forms before stirring.

Island-Style Shrimp Cocktail

SERVES 4

Per Serving

Calories	194
Fat	7g
Sodium	504mg
Carbohydrates	4g
Fiber	0g
Sugar	4g
Protein	29g

IS THE PAN HOT ENOUGH?

Hold your hand about 4" over the pan and count to three. You shouldn't be able to keep your hand comfortably over the pan for more than three seconds. Avoid using extra-virgin olive oil for this dish. The high cooking temperature may give the oil an unusual flavor.

Fresh ginger is loaded with antioxidants that can help your body fight off heart disease and promote healthy aging.

1 teaspoon minced garlic

½ teaspoon salt, divided

1 tablespoon minced fresh ginger

3 tablespoons finely chopped scallions

1 tablespoon finely chopped jalapeño pepper

¼ cup lime juice

1 tablespoon honey

1 tablespoon canola oil

1 pound extra-large (21- to 25-count) shrimp, peeled, tails left on

¼ teaspoon ground black pepper

½ medium lemon, cut into wedges

½ medium lime, cut into wedges

1 Combine garlic, ¼ teaspoon salt, ginger, scallions, jalapeño, lime juice, and honey in a small serving bowl and set aside.

2 Heat oil in a medium heavy-bottomed nonstick skillet over high heat until it starts to smoke. Season shrimp with black pepper and remaining ¼ teaspoon salt. Add shrimp to the skillet and sauté until cooked through, about 2 minutes. Remove skillet from heat and immediately add 2 tablespoons jalapeño sauce to the skillet; toss to coat shrimp.

3 Transfer shrimp to a baking sheet to cool for about 5 minutes.

4 To serve, arrange shrimp on a platter with the bowl of sauce. Garnish with lemon and lime wedges.

Soy-Glazed Tofu and Vegetable Spring Rolls

Spring rolls make a delicious light lunch, especially in warmer weather. The cool and crunchy vegetables are refreshing, and the sweet and sticky tofu adds a nice protein punch. Serve them with a sweet chili sauce for dipping.

1 (14-ounce) package extra-firm tofu, drained and pressed for 30 minutes

¼ cup cornstarch

2 tablespoons toasted sesame oil

2 tablespoons soy sauce

2 tablespoons light brown sugar

12 spring roll rice paper wrappers

6 ounces vermicelli rice noodles, cooked, drained, and rinsed

1 large carrot, peeled and julienned

1 medium red bell pepper, seeded and julienned

½ large English cucumber, julienned

1 cup chopped fresh cilantro leaves

SERVES 6	
Per Serving	
Calories	285
Fat	8g
Sodium	482mg
Carbohydrates	46g
Fiber	2g
Sugar	2g
Protein	7g

1 Slice tofu into ½"-wide rectangles and sprinkle with cornstarch. Heat oil in a large skillet over medium heat. Fry tofu until golden and crispy on both sides, about 10 minutes.

2 Whisk together soy sauce and brown sugar in a small bowl. Pour over tofu and cook until sauce thickens, 3–4 minutes, carefully stirring to coat. Remove from heat and let cool.

3 Fill a shallow dish with warm water. Dip wrappers in water for about 10 seconds, until pliable. Place wrappers on a cutting board. Top each wrapper with noodles, carrot, pepper, cucumber, cilantro, and tofu. Tuck in the sides and roll into a cylinder shape.

4 Serve immediately.

Baked Cauliflower Tots

SERVES 4

Per Serving	
Calories	256
Fat	8g
Sodium	611mg
Carbohydrates	31g
Fiber	6g
Sugar	13g
Protein	15g

Cauliflower is one of the best plant-based sources of choline, an essential nutrient that many people are deficient in. Choline is important for brain development and a healthy nervous system. One cup of cauliflower has about 10 percent of the recommended daily intake of choline.

½ large head cauliflower, cut into florets

1 cup finely-shredded Mexican cheese blend

1 large egg

¼ cup cornmeal

½ teaspoon salt

¼ teaspoon ground black pepper

½ cup ketchup or barbecue sauce

1 Preheat oven to 400° F. Spray a twenty-four-cup mini muffin tin with nonstick cooking spray. Line a large bowl with a clean kitchen towel.

2 Place cauliflower in a food processor and pulse until it resembles grains of rice. Transfer to the prepared bowl and wrap cauliflower in towel, then squeeze to remove excess moisture. Discard liquid and place cauliflower back in bowl.

3 Add cheese, egg, cornmeal, salt, and pepper to the bowl; stir to combine. Scoop the mixture by spoonfuls into the prepared muffin tin and press down firmly.

4 Bake for 15–20 minutes until golden brown.

5 Serve with ketchup for dipping.

Crispy Polenta Fries with BBQ Ketchup

Polenta is made from boiled cornmeal. You can buy it premade and wrapped in a plastic tube. This allows for transforming the polenta into all sorts of shapes and sizes. Try cutting it into rounds and frying in oil until golden.

1 (24-ounce) tube polenta

2 teaspoons extra-virgin olive oil

1 teaspoon garlic powder

1 teaspoon smoked paprika

¼ teaspoon salt

¼ teaspoon ground black pepper

½ cup ketchup

½ cup barbecue sauce

SERVES 4	
Per Serving	
Calories	203
Fat	3g
Sodium	1,131mg
Carbohydrates	41g
Fiber	0g
Sugar	12g
Protein	4g

1 Preheat oven to 450°F. Spray a large baking sheet with nonstick cooking spray or line with parchment paper.

2 Cut tube of polenta in half crosswise, then cut each half lengthwise into eight wedges.

3 Place wedges in a large bowl and toss with oil, garlic powder, paprika, salt, and pepper. Spread out evenly on the prepared baking sheet. Bake for 20–25 minutes until crispy and golden brown.

4 In a small bowl, whisk together the ketchup and barbecue sauce. Serve polenta fries with sauce.

Cherry Tomato and Basil Bruschetta

SERVES 6

Per Serving

Calories	190
Fat	10g
Sodium	303mg
Carbohydrates	22g
Fiber	1g
Sugar	1g
Protein	3g

SWITCH IT UP

Try adding chopped strawberries or blueberries to your next batch of bruschetta to increase the antioxidant and sweetness factors.

This topping keeps exceptionally well in the refrigerator for a few days. Make a large batch and enjoy a fresh bruschetta for lunch.

1 (8-ounce) French-style baguette, cut into ½" slices

4 tablespoons extra-virgin olive oil, divided

1 pint cherry tomatoes, quartered

2 cloves garlic, peeled and minced

1 small shallot, peeled and minced

1 cup packed basil leaves, thinly sliced, divided

1 teaspoon balsamic vinegar

¼ teaspoon salt

¼ teaspoon ground black pepper

1 Preheat oven to 425°F. Line a large baking sheet with parchment paper.

2 Place baguette slices on the prepared baking sheet. Brush with 2 tablespoons oil. Bake for 5 minutes, then flip and toast for another 5 minutes.

3 In a medium bowl, combine tomatoes, garlic, shallot, half of the basil, remaining 2 tablespoons oil, vinegar, salt, and pepper.

4 Place toasted bread on a serving platter and top with tomato mixture. Sprinkle remaining basil over bruschetta and serve.

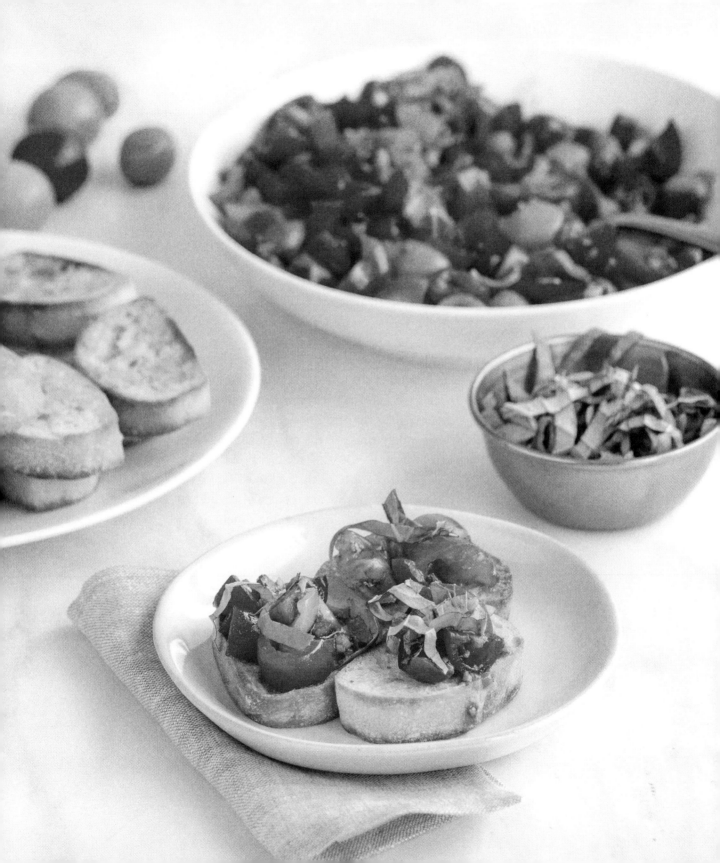

Marinated Portobello Mushrooms

SERVES 6

Per Serving

Calories	31
Fat	2g
Sodium	194mg
Carbohydrates	1g
Fiber	2g
Sugar	1g
Protein	3g

STAGES OF MUSHROOMS

Portobello mushrooms actually start out as white button mushrooms. As they mature, they turn into cremini (also called baby bella) mushrooms and then finally portobello.

Portobello mushrooms have a meaty flavor that offers a great substitute for meat in many recipes. They will boost your fiber, protein, and B vitamin intake. Mushrooms also contain the antioxidants vitamin C and selenium.

6 large portobello mushrooms

1 teaspoon extra-virgin olive oil

2 teaspoons balsamic vinegar

½ teaspoon salt

½ teaspoon cracked black pepper

¼ bunch marjoram, chopped

¼ bunch oregano, chopped

1 Remove stems from mushrooms and slice stems in half. Then scrape out and discard the black membranes.

2 In a large container, stir together oil, vinegar, salt, pepper, marjoram, and oregano. Add mushroom stems and caps and stir gently to coat. Cover and marinate in the refrigerator for at least 3 hours.

3 Preheat oven to 400°F. Place racks on two large baking sheets.

4 Place mushrooms on racks and roast for 20 minutes. Remove from oven, let mushrooms cool slightly, and cut caps into small wedges. Serve warm or at room temperature.

Curry Cayenne Peanuts

Peanuts are one of the richest sources of the vitamin biotin, which is essential for a healthy metabolism.

1 large egg white

2 tablespoons curry powder

1½ teaspoons kosher salt

1 teaspoon sugar

¼ teaspoon ground cayenne pepper

3 cups unsalted peanuts

1 Preheat oven to 300°F. Line two large baking sheets with parchment paper.

2 In a medium bowl, whisk egg white until frothy. Add curry powder, salt, sugar, and cayenne pepper; whisk until evenly blended. Add peanuts and stir until evenly coated.

3 Spread peanut mixture in a single layer on the prepared baking sheets. Roast for 20 minutes or until nuts are dry and toasted. Stir and turn the nuts at least two times during the roasting process. (Be very watchful during the last half of baking, as the nuts can burn quickly.)

4 Remove nuts from the oven and transfer them to a sheet of parchment paper to cool.

SERVES 12

Per Serving

Calories	163
Fat	13g
Sodium	245mg
Carbohydrates	5g
Fiber	2g
Sugar	1g
Protein	7g

PEA-NUTTY

Peanuts are actually not nuts at all. They are part of the legume "bean" family. They provide over thirty essential nutrients and phytochemicals. Even though peanuts are considered high in fat, they contain the good monounsaturated type of fat.

Spicy Roasted Chickpeas

SERVES 8

Per Serving

Calories	90
Fat	4g
Sodium	198mg
Carbohydrates	10g
Fiber	2g
Sugar	2g
Protein	4g

Chickpeas are a good source of fiber, containing 4 grams per ½-cup serving. Fiber helps keep us full longer between meals. Try these roasted chickpeas for a filling snack.

2 tablespoons olive oil

½ teaspoon ground coriander

½ teaspoon ground cumin

½ teaspoon crushed red pepper flakes

¼ teaspoon seasoned salt

2 cups canned chickpeas, drained and rinsed

1 Preheat oven to 400°F. Spray a large baking sheet with nonstick cooking spray.

2 In a medium bowl, combine oil, coriander, cumin, red pepper flakes, and seasoned salt. Add chickpeas and toss until evenly coated.

3 Spread coated chickpeas in a single layer on the prepared baking sheet. Bake, stirring occasionally, for 20–30 minutes until crisp and golden. Transfer chickpeas to a plate or a sheet of parchment paper to cool.

4 Serve immediately or store in an airtight container for up to 5 days.

Soups and Stews

Carrot Lemon Soup

SERVES 6

Per Serving

Calories	152
Fat	8g
Sodium	427mg
Carbohydrates	18g
Fiber	4g
Sugar	12g
Protein	2g

LEMON KNOW-HOW

The thought of lemons may make your cheeks pucker, but it's well worth it for the powerful dose of cold-fighting vitamin C they provide. The average lemon contains approximately 3 tablespoons of juice. Allow lemons to come to room temperature before squeezing to maximize the amount of juice extracted.

This soup can be served hot or cold depending on your mood. Try puréeing the soup with an immersion blender after simmering for a smooth texture.

3 tablespoons olive oil

2 pounds carrots, peeled and diced

2 large yellow onions, peeled and diced

2 cloves garlic, peeled and minced

6 cups low-sodium vegetable stock

1 teaspoon minced fresh ginger

13 tablespoons lemon juice

1 tablespoon grated lemon zest

¾ teaspoon salt

½ teaspoon ground black pepper

3 scallions, trimmed and sliced

1 Heat oil in a large stockpot or Dutch oven over medium heat. Lightly sauté carrots, onions, and garlic for 5 minutes.

2 Add stock, reduce heat to medium-low, and simmer for 1 hour. Stir in ginger, lemon juice, zest, salt, and pepper.

3 Allow soup to cool. Transfer soup to a covered container and refrigerate for at least 3 hours. Garnish with scallions before serving.

Thai Coconut Tofu Soup

Savory and full of unique and spicy flavors, this soup is sure to hit the spot. To make it totally vegan, omit the fish sauce and replace it with soy sauce to taste.

2 tablespoons olive oil

1 medium yellow onion, peeled and thinly sliced

2 tablespoons minced fresh ginger

2 cloves garlic, peeled and minced

2 tablespoons chili-garlic sauce

6 cups vegetable broth

1 (13.5-ounce) can full-fat coconut milk

1 tablespoon hoisin sauce

1 tablespoon fish sauce

1 teaspoon salt

1 medium stalk lemongrass, trimmed

1 pound white mushrooms, thinly sliced

1 (14-ounce) block firm tofu, drained, pressed, and cut into 1" pieces

2 tablespoons lime juice

1 bunch scallions, trimmed and sliced

¾ cup chopped fresh cilantro

1 cup bean sprouts

1 Heat oil in a large stockpot or Dutch oven over medium heat. Add onion, ginger, garlic, and chili-garlic sauce. Cook, stirring frequently, until onion begins to soften, 3–4 minutes.

2 Add broth, coconut milk, hoisin sauce, fish sauce, salt, and lemongrass. Bring to a boil over high heat, then reduce heat to low and simmer for 10 minutes.

3 Add mushrooms and tofu to the pot and cook for 3 minutes more.

4 Remove and discard lemongrass stalk. Stir in lime juice.

5 Divide soup among bowls and top each bowl with scallions, cilantro, and bean sprouts. Serve immediately.

SERVES 4

Per Serving	
Calories	495
Fat	36g
Sodium	882mg
Carbohydrates	29g
Fiber	5g
Sugar	12g
Protein	14g

LOVE FOR LEMONGRASS

Lemongrass stalks are light green, woody stems that look similar to scallions. You should be able to find them in the refrigerated herbs section. Lemongrass provides a lemony, gingery, and floral taste to dishes.

Gazpacho

Gazpacho is a cold Spanish soup made of blended raw vegetables. For a fun garnish, freeze good-quality olive oil in small ice cube trays. The olive oil cubes will add flavor and chill the soup.

SERVES 6

Per Serving

Calories	64
Fat	0g
Sodium	34mg
Carbohydrates	14g
Fiber	2g
Sugar	14g
Protein	2g

THE SCENT OF GARLIC

To keep your hands from smelling like garlic after you've been working with it, wash them in cold water. Hot water will seal in the garlic smell.

2 large Vidalia or other sweet onions, peeled and chopped

3 medium cucumbers, peeled and chopped

1½ pounds plum tomatoes, chopped

3 cloves garlic, peeled and minced

½ chipotle chili pepper (canned in adobo sauce)

½ bunch cilantro, stemmed and chopped

2 teaspoons grated lime zest

2 tablespoons lime juice

¼ teaspoon Tabasco sauce

½ teaspoon ground black pepper

1½ quarts low-sodium vegetable stock

1 In a large bowl, mix together all ingredients except stock. Purée all but a quarter of this mixture in a blender. (The last quarter is reserved for garnish.)

2 Add stock to the blender. Continue to purée until smooth.

3 Ladle into serving bowls and garnish with reserved vegetable mixture.

Basic Chicken Soup

Homemade chicken soup is lower in sodium than canned soup, and it can be customized to whatever vegetables you have on hand.

1 (5-pound) chicken, trimmed and quartered (reserve giblets)

12 cups water

2 medium carrots, peeled and chopped

2 stalks celery, trimmed and chopped

4 large yellow onions, peeled and chopped

¼ bunch parsley, chopped

½ teaspoon ground black pepper

¾ teaspoon kosher salt

1 Place chicken and giblets in a large stockpot or Dutch oven, add water, and bring to a boil over high heat. Reduce heat to a simmer and skim off all foam.

2 Add remaining ingredients and simmer for 3 hours, skimming foam occasionally.

3 Remove chicken and giblets from the stockpot; discard giblets. Remove meat from bones, discard bones, and return meat to broth. Serve hot.

SERVES 6

Per Serving

Calories	160
Fat	2g
Sodium	394mg
Carbohydrates	15g
Fiber	3g
Sugar	8g
Protein	23g

DON'T CRY OVER CUT ONIONS

The sulfur in onions can cause the tears to flow. To avoid teary eyes, peel onions under cold water to wash away the volatile sulfur compounds. Onions are worth the extra effort, since they have anti-inflammatory effects on the joints.

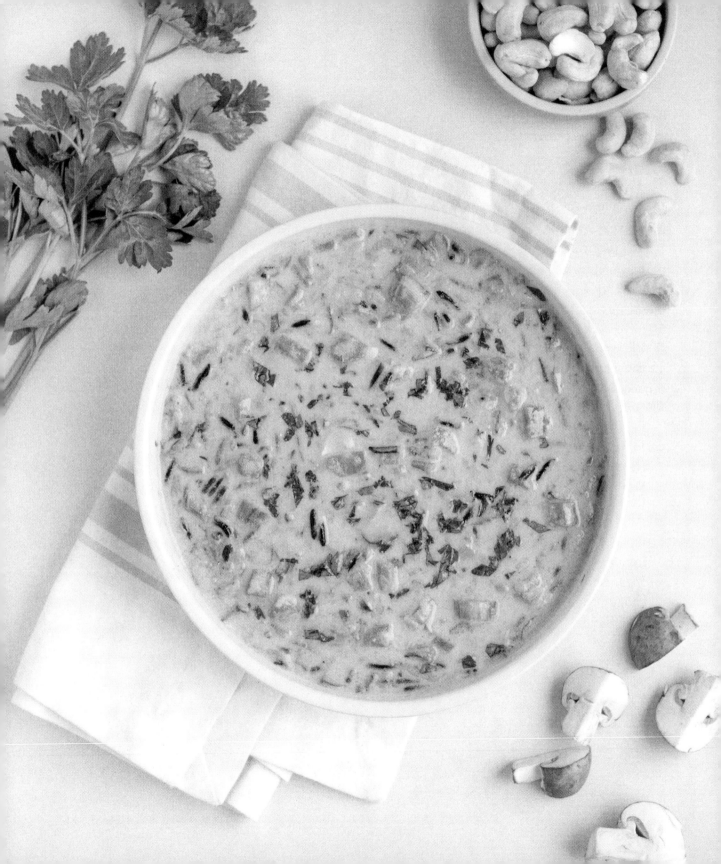

Creamy Wild Rice Soup

Wild rice is a good source of fiber, and contains the nutrient manganese, which is essential for a healthy metabolism. It's not actually a rice, but an aquatic grass that goes through a lengthy drying process to turn it into the kernels we're familiar with.

2 tablespoons extra-virgin olive oil

2 medium leeks (white and light green parts only), thinly sliced

2 cloves garlic, peeled and minced

2 medium carrots, peeled and diced

2 stalks celery, trimmed and diced

½ cup white wine

8 ounces portobello mushrooms, diced

8 ounces cremini mushrooms, diced

6 cups vegetable stock

1 cup uncooked wild rice

1 bay leaf

1 teaspoon salt

¼ teaspoon ground black pepper

1 bunch kale, stems removed and leaves chopped

1 cup raw cashews

1 cup chopped fresh Italian parsley

SERVES 4	
Per Serving	
Calories	488
Fat	21g
Sodium	700mg
Carbohydrates	53g
Fiber	10g
Sugar	15g
Protein	22g

1 Heat oil in a large stockpot or Dutch oven over medium heat. Add leeks, garlic, carrots, and celery. Cook, stirring occasionally, until tender, about 10 minutes. Add white wine and stir, scraping the bottom of the pot.

2 Add mushrooms, stock, rice, bay leaf, salt, pepper, and kale. Bring to a boil over high heat. Reduce heat to low and simmer for 30–40 minutes until rice is soft.

3 Meanwhile, place cashews in a small heatproof bowl. Add just enough boiling water to cover cashews (about 1 cup). Set aside for 15 minutes, then transfer to a blender or food processor. Purée until smooth.

4 Stir cashew cream into soup. Divide soup among bowls and top with parsley before serving.

Potato Leek Soup

SERVES 4

Per Serving

Calories	454
Fat	24g
Sodium	723mg
Carbohydrates	49g
Fiber	4g
Sugar	10g
Protein	9g

Leeks are related to chives and onions, but only the white and light green parts are edible. Trim the dark green part and discard. To clean leeks, thinly slice them and immerse in a bowl of water. Use your fingers to swish the leeks around to remove dirt, and rinse well.

2 tablespoons extra-virgin olive oil

1 medium yellow onion, peeled and diced

2 medium leeks (white and light green parts only), thinly sliced

6 medium Yukon Gold potatoes, peeled and diced

3 cloves garlic, peeled and minced

1 teaspoon dried thyme

¼ teaspoon ground coriander

½ teaspoon salt

¼ teaspoon ground black pepper

6 cups vegetable broth

2 bay leaves

1 (13.5-ounce) can full-fat coconut milk

3 tablespoons lemon juice

¼ cup finely chopped fresh chives

1 Heat oil in a large stockpot or Dutch oven over medium heat. Sauté onion and leeks until softened, 5–6 minutes.

2 Add potatoes, garlic, thyme, coriander, salt, and pepper. Cook for 3 minutes more. Add broth and bay leaves. Bring to a boil over high heat, then reduce heat to low and simmer for 20–25 minutes until potatoes are fork-tender.

3 Remove and discard bay leaves. Stir in coconut milk and lemon juice.

4 Transfer soup in batches to a blender or use an immersion blender to purée soup until smooth.

5 Top with chives before serving.

Pumpkin Soup

This is a perfect autumn soup to celebrate the harvest season. If you're short on time or if pumpkins are out of season, substitute a 15-ounce can of puréed pumpkin for the fresh pumpkin.

2 cups chopped fresh sugar pumpkin, seeds reserved separately

1 teaspoon salt, divided

3 large leeks (white and light green parts only), trimmed and sliced

1½ teaspoons minced fresh ginger

1 tablespoon light olive oil

½ teaspoon grated lemon zest

1 teaspoon lemon juice

2 quarts low-sodium vegetable stock

½ teaspoon ground black pepper

1 tablespoon extra-virgin olive oil

1. Preheat oven to 375°F. Line a large baking sheet with parchment paper.
2. Clean pumpkin seeds thoroughly and place them on the prepared baking sheet. Sprinkle with ½ teaspoon salt. Roast for 5–8 minutes until golden. Remove from oven and set aside to cool. Leave oven on.
3. In a large ungreased baking dish, combine pumpkin, leeks, ginger, and light olive oil; toss to coat. Roast for 45 minutes to 1 hour until pumpkin is tender.
4. Transfer pumpkin mixture to a large stockpot or Dutch oven and add zest, juice, stock, remaining ½ teaspoon salt, and pepper. Bring to a boil over medium-high heat, then reduce heat to medium-low. Simmer for 45 minutes.
5. Ladle soup into serving bowls. Drizzle with extra-virgin olive oil and sprinkle with toasted pumpkin seeds.

SERVES 6

Per Serving

Calories	69
Fat	4g
Sodium	409mg
Carbohydrates	7g
Fiber	1g
Sugar	4g
Protein	1g

ZESTING

If you don't have a zester, you can still easily make lemon zest. Simply use your cheese grater, but be careful to grate only the rind and not the white pith, which tends to be bitter.

Butternut Squash and Pear Soup

SERVES 6

Per Serving

Calories	208
Fat	12g
Sodium	302mg
Carbohydrates	23g
Fiber	4g
Sugar	15g
Protein	2g

A warm and comforting soup perfect for chilly weather, this is the ideal combination of sweet and savory.

3 cups diced butternut squash (about 1 small squash)

2 large ripe Bartlett pears, peeled, cored, and diced

3 tablespoons extra-virgin olive oil, divided

½ teaspoon salt

¼ teaspoon ground black pepper

2 tablespoons vegan butter

1 medium yellow onion, peeled and diced

2 cloves garlic, peeled and minced

1 teaspoon minced fresh ginger

4 cups vegetable broth

1 cup pear nectar

1 Preheat oven to 400°F.

2 In a large bowl, toss squash and pears with 2 tablespoons oil and season with salt and pepper. Spread onto a large ungreased baking sheet and roast for 25 minutes or until fork-tender.

3 Heat vegan butter and remaining 1 tablespoon oil in a large stockpot or Dutch oven over medium heat. Sauté onion, garlic, and ginger until softened, 3–4 minutes.

4 Add broth, pear nectar, and roasted squash and pears. Bring to a boil over high heat, then reduce heat to low and simmer for 5 minutes. Blend with an immersion blender or transfer to a regular blender in batches and process until smooth.

5 Serve hot.

Split Pea Soup

Peas and other legumes are good sources of fiber and protein in vegetarian diets. To make this meal completely vegetarian, omit the ham bone and use vegetable stock in place of the water.

8 cups water

2 cups split peas

1 ham bone

½ cup diced carrot

¼ cup diced celery

1 cup diced yellow onion

¾ teaspoon salt

½ teaspoon ground black pepper

SERVES 6	
Per Serving	
Calories	238
Fat	10g
Sodium	1,110mg
Carbohydrates	16g
Fiber	6g
Sugar	3g
Protein	21g

1 In a large stockpot or Dutch oven, combine water, split peas, and ham bone. Bring to a boil over high heat, then reduce heat to medium-low and simmer for 1 hour.

2 Add carrot, celery, and onion and simmer for 1 hour.

3 Remove ham bone and season soup with salt and pepper. Serve hot.

Tortilla Soup

This vibrant soup is full of healthy fiber and flavor from beans and peppers. The tortillas soften in the broth and have a dumpling-like texture.

2 tablespoons extra-virgin olive oil

1 medium yellow onion, peeled and diced

1 teaspoon chili powder

1 teaspoon salt

½ teaspoon paprika

¼ teaspoon ground black pepper

1 (4-ounce) can green chilies

1 medium red bell pepper, seeded and diced

1 (15-ounce) can black beans, drained and rinsed

1 (15-ounce) can kidney beans, drained and rinsed

1 (15-ounce) can corn kernels

6 cups vegetable broth

1 (15-ounce) can tomato sauce

4 (6") flour tortillas, cut into strips

1 cup chopped fresh cilantro leaves

1 large avocado, peeled, pitted, and sliced

⅓ cup vegan sour cream

¾ cup shredded vegan Cheddar-style cheese

1 Heat oil in a large stockpot or Dutch oven over medium heat. Add onion, chili powder, salt, paprika, and black pepper and cook, stirring occasionally, until onion begins to soften, 3–4 minutes.

2 Add chilies, bell pepper, beans, corn, broth, and tomato sauce. Bring to a boil over high heat, then reduce heat to low and simmer for 30 minutes.

3 Divide soup among bowls. Stir in tortilla strips. Top with cilantro, avocado, vegan sour cream, and vegan cheese.

Roasted Root Vegetable Soup

Root vegetables such as carrots, parsnips, and sweet potatoes are loaded with anti-inflammatory nutrients. Onions are also rich in the antioxidant compounds flavonoids, and are a great prebiotic to help healthy gut bacteria thrive.

1 tablespoon olive oil

2 large parsnips, peeled and chopped

3 large carrots, peeled and chopped

2 medium sweet potatoes, peeled and chopped

3 stalks celery, trimmed and chopped

3 medium yellow onions, peeled and cut into wedges

1 sprig fresh rosemary

4 cups low-sodium vegetable stock

3 sprigs fresh thyme, stemmed and chopped

¼ bunch fresh parsley, stemmed and chopped

2 bay leaves

½ teaspoon ground black pepper

¾ teaspoon salt

1. Preheat oven to 375°F.
2. Pour oil into a large roasting pan. Place parsnips, carrots, sweet potatoes, celery, onions, and rosemary sprig in the pan and roast until tender, 30–45 minutes. Remove from oven, discard rosemary sprig, and let cool slightly.
3. In a blender or food processor, purée roasted vegetables thoroughly in small batches. Add stock to the blender as needed to create a smooth mixture. Pour the mixture into a large stockpot or Dutch oven with the remaining stock and bring to a simmer over medium heat.
4. Add thyme, parsley, bay leaves, pepper, and salt to the pot and continue to simmer for 1 hour. Remove and discard bay leaves. Serve hot.

SERVES 6	
Per Serving	
Calories	121
Fat	3g
Sodium	363mg
Carbohydrates	22g
Fiber	5g
Sugar	12g
Protein	2g

EVERGREEN TO THE RESCUE

Rosemary is the disease-fighting product of an evergreen tree. It has a wonderful pine-like fragrance and a pungent taste that can give chicken, pork, fish, and soups a major flavor boost. It also offers anti-inflammatory qualities that may reduce the severity of asthma attacks.

Minestrone

SERVES 6

Per Serving

Calories	358
Fat	16g
Sodium	623mg
Carbohydrates	28g
Fiber	7g
Sugar	10g
Protein	26g

PINING FOR NUTS

Pine nuts are a wonderful addition to soups, sauces, and other dishes. They offer healthy fats, as well as numerous vitamins and minerals with antioxidant benefits. Raw pine nuts should be refrigerated to maintain freshness.

An ideal entrée for cool, crisp fall days, this soup is chock-full of vegetables and lean sources of protein such as turkey sausage and beans.

1 teaspoon olive oil

1 pound Italian turkey sausage, thinly sliced

1 medium bulb fennel, trimmed and roughly chopped

1 large leek (white and light green parts only), trimmed and thinly sliced

1 medium yellow onion, peeled and sliced

1 medium shallot, peeled and sliced

4 cloves garlic, peeled and minced

½ head savoy cabbage

8 medium plum tomatoes, roughly chopped

1 cup dry red wine

2 quarts low-sodium vegetable stock

½ teaspoon ground black pepper

4 sprigs fresh marjoram, stemmed and chopped

2 sprigs fresh oregano, stemmed and chopped

¼ bunch fresh basil, stemmed and chopped

1 cup cooked cannellini beans

1 cup small pasta, cooked al dente and drained

¼ cup toasted pine nuts

2 ounces grated Romano cheese

2 ounces grated Parmesan cheese

1 Heat oil in a large stockpot or Dutch oven over medium heat. Add sausage, fennel, leek, onion, shallot, garlic, cabbage, and tomatoes; sauté for 8–10 minutes until vegetables soften.

2 Add wine and cook, stirring occasionally, until reduced by half, about 5 minutes. Stir in stock, pepper, marjoram, oregano, and basil; reduce heat to low and simmer for 4 hours.

3 Add beans and pasta; cook for 8 minutes.

4 Serve with pine nuts and cheeses sprinkled over the top.

Spinach and Mushroom Lasagna Soup

What's better than a baked lasagna? Lasagna in a bowl made with plant-based ingredients! Try this delicious version of lasagna made in a soup pot on a cold winter night.

2 tablespoons extra-virgin olive oil, divided

1 medium yellow onion, peeled and diced

8 ounces cremini mushrooms, thinly sliced

2 cloves garlic, peeled and minced

1 (24-ounce) jar marinara sauce

3 cups vegetable broth

1 (14.5-ounce) can diced tomatoes

2 tablespoons tomato paste

2 teaspoons balsamic vinegar

1 tablespoon dried basil

1 teaspoon dried oregano

½ teaspoon salt

½ teaspoon ground black pepper

1 bay leaf

6 lasagna noodles, broken into pieces

12 ounces vegan crumbles (ground meat substitute)

5 ounces baby spinach

½ cup vegan ricotta

1 cup shredded vegan mozzarella-style cheese

SERVES 4

Per Serving

Calories	654
Fat	27g
Sodium	620mg
Carbohydrates	69g
Fiber	10g
Sugar	12g
Protein	29g

1 Heat 1 tablespoon oil in a large stockpot or Dutch oven over medium heat. Sauté onion and mushrooms until softened, 5–7 minutes. Add garlic and sauté 1 minute.

2 Add marinara sauce, broth, tomatoes, tomato paste, vinegar, basil, oregano, salt, pepper, and bay leaf. Bring to a boil over high heat, then reduce heat to low. Add lasagna noodles and simmer, stirring often, until noodles are softened, about 15 minutes.

3 Meanwhile, heat remaining 1 tablespoon oil in a medium non-stick skillet over medium-high heat. Add vegan crumbles and sauté until browned, about 10 minutes. Remove from heat and set aside.

4 When lasagna noodles are soft, add vegan crumbles and spinach to soup and stir until spinach is wilted.

5 Remove and discard bay leaf. Serve soup with a dollop of vegan ricotta and a sprinkle of shredded vegan cheese.

Wedding Soup

SERVES 6

Per Serving

Calories	226
Fat	10g
Sodium	505mg
Carbohydrates	13g
Fiber	1g
Sugar	1g
Protein	21g

This soup is full of ingredients—parsley, oregano, basil, and spinach—that are known for their antioxidant and anti-inflammatory properties.

3 (1-ounce) slices Italian bread, toasted

¾ pound lean ground beef

1 large egg or ¼ cup egg substitute

1 medium yellow onion, peeled and chopped

3 cloves garlic, peeled and minced

¼ bunch fresh parsley, stemmed and chopped

3 sprigs fresh oregano, stemmed and chopped

2 sprigs fresh basil, stemmed and chopped

½ teaspoon ground black pepper

½ cup grated Parmesan cheese, divided

2 quarts low-sodium chicken stock

1 cup roughly chopped fresh baby spinach

1 Preheat oven to 375°F.

2 Place bread in a large bowl and wet with a bit of water. Squeeze out liquid and return soaked bread to the bowl.

3 Add ground beef, egg, onion, garlic, parsley, oregano, basil, pepper, and ¼ cup Parmesan cheese. Form mixture into 1" balls and place in a medium ungreased baking dish. Bake meatballs for 20 minutes. Remove from oven and drain on paper towels.

4 In a large stockpot or Dutch oven, combine stock, spinach, and meatballs. Bring to a boil over high heat. Reduce heat to medium-low and simmer for 30 minutes.

5 Ladle soup into serving bowls and sprinkle with remaining cheese before serving.

Mediterranean Stew

Full of plant-based protein and fiber from two types of beans, this soup is sure to fill you up! Serve with warmed pita bread.

3 tablespoons olive oil

3 cloves garlic, peeled and minced

1 (15-ounce) can chickpeas, drained and rinsed

1 (15-ounce) can cannellini beans, drained and rinsed

2 cups diced tomatoes

1½ cups artichoke hearts, quartered

1 cup low-sodium vegetable stock

4 tablespoons grated Parmesan cheese

1 teaspoon crushed red pepper flakes

1 teaspoon dried oregano

½ teaspoon salt

½ teaspoon ground black pepper

½ cup chopped sun-dried tomatoes

1 cup garlic-seasoned croutons

½ cup crumbled feta cheese

1 tablespoon fresh oregano leaves

½ cup chopped fresh Italian parsley

SERVES 4	
Per Serving	
Calories	681
Fat	21g
Sodium	563mg
Carbohydrates	88g
Fiber	25g
Sugar	18g
Protein	35g

1 Heat oil in a large stockpot or Dutch oven over medium heat and sauté garlic for 1–2 minutes until golden.

2 Reduce heat to medium-low. Stir in chickpeas, cannellini beans, diced tomatoes, artichoke hearts, stock, Parmesan cheese, crushed red pepper flakes, oregano, salt, and black pepper. Cook, stirring occasionally, for 10 minutes.

3 Ladle soup into four bowls and top each with sun-dried tomatoes, croutons, feta cheese, oregano, and parsley. Serve immediately.

Bean and Lentil Ragout

A ragout is typically a dish containing highly seasoned meat cut into small pieces, stewed with vegetables. In this version, the meat is replaced with beans and lentils for a hearty plant-based dish full of inflammation-fighting ingredients.

SERVES 6

Per Serving

Calories	164
Fat	5g
Sodium	90mg
Carbohydrates	22g
Fiber	7g
Sugar	9g
Protein	7g

BENEFITS OF BEANS

Beans are an excellent source of eight of the nine essential amino acids necessary for the formation of a variety of proteins in the body. They also pack a powerful fiber punch with 9–13 grams of fiber per cup. Their protein-fiber combination will keep hunger at bay for hours.

2 tablespoons olive oil

1 large yellow onion, peeled and finely diced

1 stalk celery, trimmed and finely diced

½ large leek (white and light green parts only), trimmed and finely diced

1 large carrot, peeled and finely diced

3 cloves garlic, peeled and minced

6 medium tomatoes, diced

½ cup cooked cannellini beans

¼ cup dried red lentils

¼ cup dried yellow lentils

2 sprigs fresh thyme, stemmed and chopped

¼ bunch fresh parsley, stemmed and chopped

2 bay leaves

½ teaspoon ground cinnamon

½ teaspoon ground turmeric or curry powder

½ teaspoon chili powder

½ teaspoon ground cumin

1 quart low-sodium vegetable stock

1 Heat oil in a large stockpot or Dutch oven over medium heat. Put in onion, celery, leek, carrot, and garlic; sauté for 2 minutes. Add tomatoes, beans, and lentils; sauté for 1 minute.

2 Add thyme, parsley, bay leaves, cinnamon, turmeric, chili powder, and cumin; stir for 1 minute, then add stock. Reduce heat to medium-low and simmer for 1 hour. Remove and discard bay leaves. Serve hot.

Chickpea Stew

Dried beans are more economical than canned, but you'll need to start this recipe one day in advance. Salting the eggplant helps remove the bitter flavor before cooking.

1 cup dried chickpeas

1 large eggplant, trimmed and diced

2 teaspoons kosher salt

3 tablespoons olive oil

1 medium yellow onion, peeled and chopped

3 cloves garlic, peeled and minced

4 medium tomatoes, peeled and chopped

1 large potato, diced

1 large zucchini, trimmed and diced

1 teaspoon fennel seeds, crushed

1 cup low-sodium vegetable stock

½ teaspoon table salt

½ teaspoon ground black pepper

SERVES 6	
Per Serving	
Calories	197
Fat	7g
Sodium	21mg
Carbohydrates	28g
Fiber	7g
Sugar	8g
Protein	6g

1 Place chickpeas in a medium bowl and cover with water. Soak overnight; drain and rinse.

2 Place eggplant in a colander and sprinkle with kosher salt. Cover with a paper towel and set aside for 30 minutes, then rinse and pat dry.

3 Heat oil in a large stockpot or Dutch oven over medium heat. Sauté onion until softened, 3–4 minutes. Add garlic and sauté for 30 seconds. Add eggplant and sauté lightly until it becomes golden, about 8 minutes.

4 Add tomatoes, potato, zucchini, fennel seeds, chickpeas, stock, table salt, and pepper. Increase heat to high and bring to a boil. Cover, reduce heat to medium-low, and simmer for 30 minutes or until chickpeas are tender. Serve hot.

Spicy Seafood Stew

SERVES 6

Per Serving

Calories	190
Fat	6g
Sodium	643mg
Carbohydrates	9g
Fiber	2g
Sugar	4g
Protein	25g

FISH STORAGE FACTS

If you're unable to cook fresh fish on the day it is purchased, store the fish on a bed of ice in the coldest part of the refrigerator. The same applies for shellfish.

Wild-caught salmon is a smart choice for this delicious soup. Salmon is a great source of protein, heart-healthy fats, and vitamin B_{12}, which is essential for a healthy metabolism and nerves.

2 tablespoons olive oil

½ cup chopped yellow onion

½ cup diced green bell pepper

1 tablespoon minced garlic

3 cups canned diced tomatoes, undrained

½ cup coconut milk

1 teaspoon hot pepper sauce

¼ cup freshly squeezed lime juice

½ teaspoon seasoned salt

¾ pound skinless firm-fleshed fish fillets, such as center-cut salmon, cod, or halibut

¾ pound medium shrimp, shelled and deveined

½ cup thinly sliced scallions

½ cup chopped fresh cilantro

1 Heat oil in a large skillet over medium-high heat. Add onion, green pepper, garlic, and tomatoes. Bring to a simmer, stirring occasionally, and cook until vegetables begin to soften, 3–4 minutes.

2 Add coconut milk, pepper sauce, lime juice, and seasoned salt. Bring to a simmer and cook for 2 minutes. Add fish and stir, being careful not to break apart the fillets. Cook until fish is cooked through and flakes easily, about 8 minutes. Add shrimp and cook until opaque and cooked through, about 3 minutes.

3 Use a slotted spoon to transfer equal amounts of fish and shrimp to six shallow serving bowls. Pour sauce over seafood and garnish with scallions and cilantro. Serve hot.

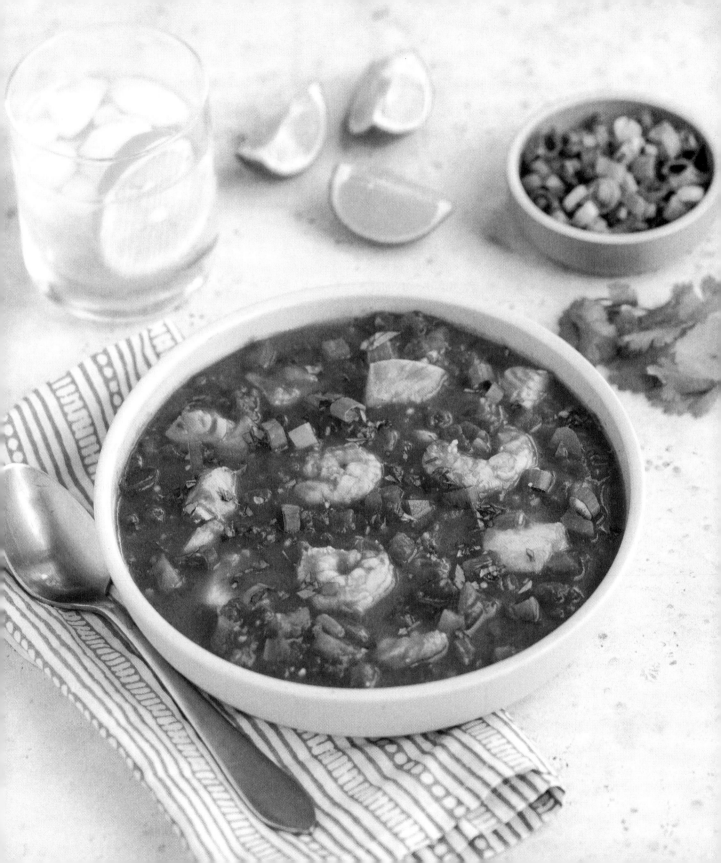

Harvest Vegetable and Beef Stew

SERVES 6

Per Serving

Calories	229
Fat	8g
Sodium	648mg
Carbohydrates	20g
Fiber	4g
Sugar	7g
Protein	19g

Add fresh herbs from your garden to this soup, and throw in any vegetables you may have on hand. Stir in chopped spinach or kale before serving to ramp up the antioxidants.

2 tablespoons olive oil

1 pound stewing beef, cut into 1" cubes

¼ cup all-purpose flour

¾ cup diced yellow onion

½ cup sliced carrots

½ cup diced celery

1 large leek (white and light green parts only), trimmed and diced

6 cloves garlic, peeled and minced

2 cups diced zucchini

1 medium potato, peeled and diced

3 medium turnips, trimmed and diced

2 large tomatoes, chopped

1 bay leaf

3 sprigs fresh thyme

4 cups low-sodium beef broth

2 tablespoons Worcestershire sauce

½ teaspoon salt

½ teaspoon ground black pepper

1 Heat oil in a large stockpot or Dutch oven over medium-high heat. Brown beef cubes for 8 minutes, turning often. Sprinkle flour over meat and stir to coat and distribute.

2 Add onion, carrots, celery, leek, garlic, zucchini, potato, turnips, tomatoes, bay leaf, thyme sprigs, and beef broth. Bring to a boil, then reduce heat to low and simmer for 1 hour.

3 Remove and discard bay leaf and thyme sprigs. Add Worcestershire sauce, salt, and pepper and stir. Serve hot.

Black Bean Chili

A unique take on chili, this delicious dish contains whole-grain brown rice for added fiber and chopped fresh pineapple for sweetness.

1½ cups dried black beans

2 tablespoons canola oil

2 large sweet onions, peeled and chopped

5 cloves garlic, peeled and minced

1 tablespoon ground cumin

1 tablespoon dried oregano

3 tablespoons salt-free chili powder

1 teaspoon ground black pepper

1 teaspoon crushed red pepper flakes

1 teaspoon dried lemon granules, crushed

3 small jalapeño peppers, seeded and minced

2 (14.5-ounce) cans no-salt-added diced tomatoes

1 cup chopped fresh pineapple

4 large carrots, peeled and sliced

1 cup uncooked long-grain brown rice

1 tablespoon apple cider or red wine vinegar

¾ cup chopped fresh cilantro

SERVES 8	
Per Serving	
Calories	218
Fat	4g
Sodium	119mg
Carbohydrates	38g
Fiber	7g
Sugar	7g
Protein	7g

CHILI POWDERS

Using a combination of chili powders such as ancho, chipotle, or specialty salt-free chili powder blends in Black Bean Chili is an easy way to add layers of flavor. You can also substitute chunk pineapple canned in its own juice if fresh pineapple isn't available, or substitute 1 cup of fresh orange juice instead.

1 Rinse beans and place in a large heavy pot. Add water to the pot until beans are covered. Bring to a boil over medium-high heat. Drain and rinse again. Return beans to pot and add 7 cups water. Bring to a boil over medium-high heat. Reduce heat to low and simmer for 1 hour.

2 Meanwhile, heat oil in a large skillet over medium heat. Sauté onions until softened, 3–4 minutes. Add garlic and sauté for 30 seconds. Reduce heat to medium-low.

3 Stir in cumin, oregano, chili powder, black pepper, crushed red pepper flakes, lemon granules, and jalapeños. Sauté for 4 minutes, then add tomatoes. Simmer for 10 minutes, stirring frequently.

4 Stir tomato mixture into the pot of beans. Add pineapple, carrots, and rice. Simmer, partially covered, over medium-low heat for 1 hour or until beans are soft and rice is done.

5 Remove from heat and stir in vinegar. Garnish with cilantro before serving.

Lentil and Walnut Chili

SERVES 6

Per Serving

Calories	385
Fat	9g
Sodium	38mg
Carbohydrates	55g
Fiber	21g
Sugar	11g
Protein	21g

IT'S NOT HOT, IT'S CHILI

Fruity, smoky, citrusy, woodsy...these are just a few words to describe the flavors of various chilies. Make dried chilies ready for use by toasting them in a 350°F oven for 5 minutes or until they soften, become fragrant, and smoke lightly. Then soak them in enough water to cover for 1 hour, and purée in a blender with just enough soaking liquid to make a thick purée circulate in the blender. For less "heat," remove the seeds before soaking.

The star of this dish, the poblano chili, is a large chili pepper originating from Mexico that is mildly spicy. If you can't find them fresh, substitute a small can of green chilies.

1 tablespoon olive oil

2 medium shallots, peeled and sliced

4 cloves garlic, peeled and minced

2 medium poblano chilies, seeded and diced

1½ cups low-sodium vegetable stock

2½ cups canned low-sodium tomato sauce

½ cup finely chopped walnuts

1 teaspoon ground cumin

1½ tablespoons chili powder

1 tablespoon honey

2 cups dried red lentils

½ cup nonfat plain yogurt

1 Heat oil in a large stockpot or Dutch oven over medium heat. Add shallots, garlic, and poblano chilies; sauté for 2 minutes.

2 Add stock, tomato sauce, walnuts, cumin, chili powder, and honey. Bring to a boil, then reduce heat to medium-low and simmer for 1 hour. Add lentils and cook for 30 minutes longer.

3 Ladle chili into bowls. Serve with a dollop of yogurt.

Asian Soy Chili

Black bean–garlic paste is made from fermented black soybeans and garlic. It adds a sweet and salty component to this unusual chili.

3 tablespoons canola oil

1 large yellow onion, peeled and diced

1½ tablespoons minced garlic

1½ tablespoons minced fresh ginger

1 tablespoon black bean–garlic paste

6 ounces vegan crumbles (ground meat substitute)

1 (10-ounce) package frozen shelled edamame, thawed

1 cup crumbled firm tofu

1 cup vegetable broth

1 tablespoon soy sauce

1 teaspoon toasted sesame oil

1 teaspoon crushed red pepper flakes

1 Heat oil in a large stockpot or Dutch oven over medium heat and sauté onion, garlic, and ginger for 2–3 minutes until fragrant. Stir in black bean–garlic paste and vegan crumbles. Sauté for 4 minutes.

2 Reduce heat to medium-low. Stir in edamame, tofu, broth, soy sauce, sesame oil, and crushed red pepper flakes. Cook, stirring occasionally, for 10 minutes. Serve hot.

SERVES 4

Per Serving

Calories	311
Fat	18g
Sodium	453mg
Carbohydrates	19g
Fiber	2g
Sugar	3g
Protein	18g

THE TASTE OF TOFU

Tofu has very little taste on its own. It relies on seasoning and marinades to bring out its true colors. Therefore, tofu can be adapted to any type of dish imaginable. Its presence will give the dish a powerful protein and phytochemical infusion.

CHAPTER 5

Vegetables and Greens

Citrus-Steamed Carrots

Carrots are an excellent source of vitamin A, which is essential for healthy vision and the immune system. It also helps the heart and lungs work properly.

1 cup orange juice

2 tablespoons lemon juice

2 tablespoons lime juice

1 pound carrots, peeled and julienned

½ teaspoon salt

1 In a large saucepan over medium-high heat, combine orange, lemon, and lime juices. Add carrots, cover, and cook until just tender, about 5 minutes.

2 Season with salt before serving.

Parmesan-Roasted Broccoli

Roasting broccoli at a high temperature brings out its sweetness and eliminates some of the bitterness. Topping it with salty Parmesan takes it to the next level!

3 large heads broccoli, trimmed and cut into florets

3 tablespoons olive oil

2 cloves garlic, peeled and minced

½ teaspoon salt

¼ teaspoon ground black pepper

3 tablespoons lemon juice

½ cup shaved Parmesan cheese

1 Preheat oven to 400°F. Line a large baking sheet with parchment paper.
2 In a large bowl, toss broccoli with oil, garlic, salt, and pepper. Spread out in an even layer on the prepared baking sheet. Roast for 20 minutes or until broccoli begins to brown.
3 Remove from oven and top with lemon juice and Parmesan. Serve immediately.

SERVES 6

Per Serving

Calories	111
Fat	9g
Sodium	360mg
Carbohydrates	4g
Fiber	1g
Sugar	1g
Protein	4g

Roasted Peppers

Besides broiling, you can also grill peppers over a gas grill or stove-top. Hold peppers over the open flame with tongs and turn often until blistered on all sides. Then follow the same ice bath directions in this recipe.

SERVES 6

Per Serving

Calories	65
Fat	4g
Sodium	234mg
Carbohydrates	6g
Fiber	2g
Sugar	0g
Protein	1g

ROASTED PEPPER USES

Roasted peppers can be enjoyed in a variety of ways. Eat them plain with salt and pepper. Toss with cooked pasta and Parmesan. Slice and add to sandwiches.

2 tablespoons olive oil

2 large green bell peppers

2 large yellow bell peppers

2 large red bell peppers

6 cloves garlic, peeled and minced

½ teaspoon salt

½ teaspoon ground black pepper

1 Preheat broiler. Have on hand a large bowl filled with ice and water.

2 Pour oil into a stainless steel bowl. Dip bell peppers one at a time in oil and turn to coat. Reserve any remaining oil in the bowl.

3 Place bell peppers on a large ungreased baking sheet. Broil, turning often, 7–10 minutes until evenly blackened.

4 Plunge bell peppers in the ice water and set aside for 5 minutes.

5 Remove bell peppers from water, blot dry, and cut each in quarters. Peel and seed quarters, then cut into thin slices.

6 Add bell pepper slices to reserved oil, along with garlic, salt, and black pepper. Stir to combine.

7 Let sit at room temperature for at least 30 minutes before serving.

Lemon Rosemary Green Beans

Rosemary is rich in antioxidants and anti-inflammatory compounds. It is thought to help the immune system fight off disease, improve memory and cognitive function, and increase alertness and focus.

1 tablespoon plus ½ teaspoon salt, divided

1 pound fresh green beans, ends trimmed, cut into 1" pieces

2 teaspoons minced fresh rosemary

1 teaspoon grated lemon zest

1 tablespoon olive oil

½ teaspoon ground black pepper

SERVES 4	
Per Serving	
Calories	65
Fat	4g
Sodium	298mg
Carbohydrates	6g
Fiber	3g
Sugar	4g
Protein	1g

1　Fill a medium saucepan with cold water and add 1 tablespoon salt. Bring to a boil over high heat. Add beans and cook until they are a vibrant green, about 4 minutes.

2　Drain beans and transfer to a large bowl. Add rosemary, zest, oil, pepper, and remaining ½ teaspoon salt. Toss to coat evenly. Serve warm or at room temperature.

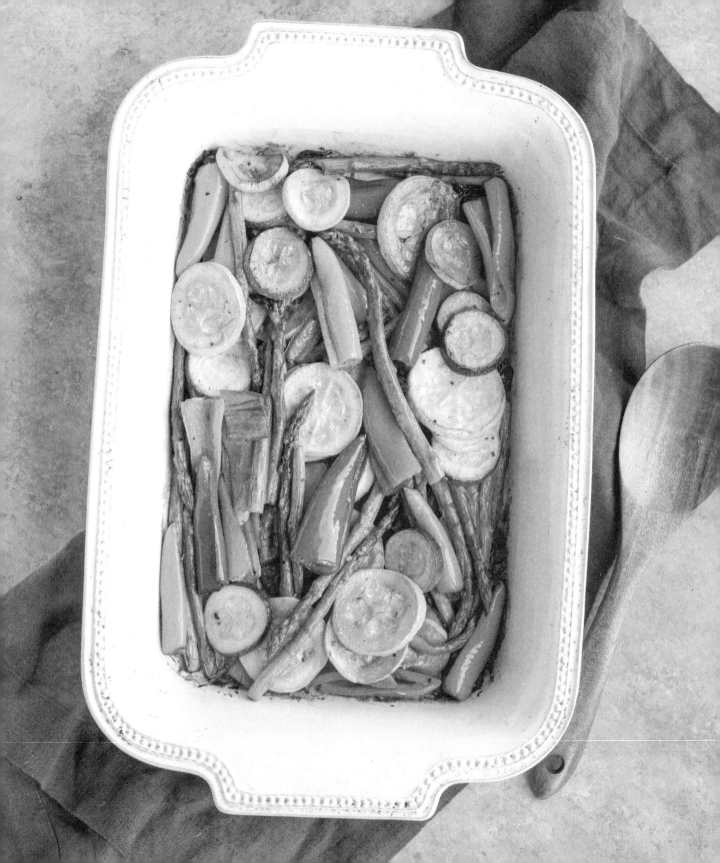

Roasted Asparagus with Summer Squash and Peppers

Asparagus is high in the antioxidant quercetin, which is known to have blood pressure–lowering and anti-inflammatory effects.

¼ cup olive oil

3 tablespoons balsamic vinegar

1 tablespoon minced garlic

1 pound asparagus, trimmed

½ pound yellow summer squash, trimmed and thinly sliced

½ pound zucchini, trimmed and thinly sliced

1 pound mini sweet peppers, seeded and sliced in half lengthwise

2 small jalapeño peppers, seeded and chopped

½ teaspoon seasoned salt

1 Preheat oven to 400°F.
2 In a small bowl, mix together oil, vinegar, and garlic and set aside.
3 Place vegetables in a large ungreased roasting pan, mixing them together. Pour oil mixture over vegetables and toss to coat. Sprinkle vegetables with seasoned salt.
4 Roast vegetables for 45 minutes or until they begin to darken; stir occasionally. Serve hot.

SERVES 4

Per Serving

Calories	227
Fat	13g
Sodium	206mg
Carbohydrates	21g
Fiber	9g
Sugar	9g
Protein	6g

ALL ABOUT BALSAMIC

Balsamic vinegar is a very dark and concentrated vinegar made from crushed and fermented grapes, seeds, and stems. The thicker, darker, and more syrup-like the vinegar is, the higher the quality.

Baked Acorn Squash

SERVES 6

Per Serving

Calories	89
Fat	0g
Sodium	293mg
Carbohydrates	21g
Fiber	3g
Sugar	0g
Protein	1g

SEASON THE SEEDS

To make a great garnish for this dish, season the squash seeds with some salt, pepper, and curry powder, then toast them in the oven or on the stovetop.

Although known as a winter squash, acorn squash can be found any time of the year. It has a dark green outer skin with longitudinal ridges, with a sweet yellow flesh inside.

3 medium acorn squash, halved and seeded

1 cup low-sodium chicken stock

1 teaspoon curry powder

½ teaspoon salt

½ teaspoon ground black pepper

1 Preheat oven to 350°F.

2 Place squash halves (cut side up) in a large ungreased baking dish. Pour stock into the bottom of the baking dish. Sprinkle squash with curry powder, salt, and pepper. Cover and bake for 45 minutes.

3 Uncover, baste squash with pan juices, and bake uncovered for another 15 minutes or until fork-tender. Serve hot.

Oven-Steamed Spaghetti Squash

Spaghetti squash is aptly named—its sweet and toothsome strands resemble spaghetti noodles. Try tossing cooked spaghetti squash strands with your favorite jarred marinara sauce.

2 large spaghetti squash, halved and seeded

1 cup water

¼ cup olive oil

½ teaspoon ground black pepper

1. Preheat oven to 350°F.
2. Place squash halves (cut side up) in a large ungreased baking dish. Pour water into the bottom of the baking dish. Cover and bake for 45–60 minutes until fork-tender.
3. Remove from oven and let cool slightly. Scrape out the insides of squash halves, spooning the flesh into a serving bowl. Drizzle with olive oil and sprinkle with pepper before serving.

SERVES 6

Per Serving

Calories	166
Fat	8g
Sodium	58mg
Carbohydrates	21g
Fiber	4g
Sugar	8g
Protein	2g

OVEN STEAMING

Oven steaming is a convenient method of healthy food preparation without the hassle of having to watch over a pot on top of the stove.

Spaghetti Squash Pancakes

SERVES 4

Per Serving

Calories	278
Fat	14g
Sodium	387mg
Carbohydrates	30g
Fiber	5g
Sugar	1g
Protein	8g

Spaghetti squash makes delicious fritters. Serve these as a side dish or with a vegetable-rich sauce and grated Parmesan on top.

1 Oven-Steamed Spaghetti Squash (see recipe in this chapter), prepared without olive oil and ground black pepper, cooled enough to handle

½ cup all-purpose flour

½ cup grated Parmesan cheese

1 large egg, beaten

2 cloves garlic, peeled and minced

¼ teaspoon salt

¼ teaspoon ground black pepper

2 tablespoons extra-virgin olive oil

¼ cup sour cream

2 scallions, trimmed and thinly sliced

1 With clean hands, squeeze squash over a colander in the sink to remove as much water as possible. Place squash in a large bowl.

2 Add flour, Parmesan, egg, garlic, salt, and pepper and stir to combine.

3 Heat oil in a large skillet over medium-high heat. Using a ¼-cup measure, scoop four portions of the squash mixture into the hot skillet and flatten with a spatula. Fry pancakes for 5–6 minutes per side until browned. Transfer to a paper towel–lined plate. Repeat with remaining squash mixture.

4 Top pancakes with sour cream and scallions before serving.

Grilled Asparagus

Asparagus provides numerous vitamins and minerals, most notably folate and potassium. The stalks also offer a blast of inflammation-fighting antioxidants.

2 bunches asparagus, trimmed

1 tablespoon extra-virgin olive oil

¾ teaspoon salt

½ teaspoon ground black pepper

1 Preheat a charcoal or gas grill.

2 In a large bowl, toss asparagus with oil, then transfer to a platter and season with salt and pepper.

3 Grill asparagus for 1–2 minutes on each side until crisp-tender and lightly browned. Serve hot or at room temperature.

SERVES 6

Per Serving

Calories	57
Fat	2g
Sodium	291mg
Carbohydrates	7g
Fiber	4g
Sugar	3g
Protein	3g

STORING ASPARAGUS

To store asparagus, trim off the bottom 1″ of stalks and discard. Place asparagus stalks in a large Mason jar and fill with 1″ water. Cover jar with a plastic bag and secure with a rubber band. This will keep asparagus crisp and fresh in the refrigerator for up to a week.

Grilled Vegetable Kebabs

SERVES 6

Per Serving

Calories	57
Fat	2g
Sodium	201mg
Carbohydrates	8g
Fiber	2g
Sugar	4g
Protein	2g

SOAKING THE SKEWERS

When using wooden skewers in cooking, always soak them in water for at least 30 minutes before spearing the food items. Soaking the skewers allows you to place them on the grill for a time without them burning.

Did you know that all bell peppers start out green? As they ripen on the vine, they turn yellow, then orange, and finally red. Bell peppers are very high in vitamin C, making them one of the best vegetable sources of this important nutrient.

1 large red onion, peeled and cut into wedges

1 large red bell pepper, seeded and cut into large chunks

1 large yellow bell pepper, seeded and cut into large chunks

1 large green bell pepper, seeded and cut into large chunks

12 large button mushrooms

1 tablespoon olive oil

½ teaspoon salt

½ teaspoon ground black pepper

1 Cut twelve standard wooden skewers in half, then soak them in water for at least 1 hour.

2 Preheat grill or broiler.

3 Thread onion, bell peppers, and mushrooms onto the skewers and brush all sides of vegetables with oil. Season with salt and black pepper.

4 Place skewers on the grill or under the broiler, paying close attention as they cook (they can easily burn). Cook until the vegetables are fork-tender, 8–10 minutes. Serve.

Roasted Potatoes with Vegetables

Serve these delicious root vegetables as a side dish, or top with fried eggs and avocado for a delicious breakfast.

3 large baking potatoes, roughly chopped

1 large sweet potato, roughly chopped

3 medium carrots, peeled and roughly chopped

1 large yellow onion, peeled and roughly chopped

½ pound button mushrooms

2 tablespoons olive oil

¾ teaspoon salt

½ teaspoon ground black pepper

1 Preheat oven to 400°F.

2 In a large bowl, mix together potatoes, carrots, onion, mushrooms, and oil. Transfer to a large ungreased roasting pan and sprinkle with salt and pepper.

3 Roast for 30–45 minutes until tender. Serve warm.

SERVES 6

Per Serving

Calories	266
Fat	6g
Sodium	362mg
Carbohydrates	47g
Fiber	5g
Sugar	6g
Protein	6g

Maple-Roasted Butternut Squash and Brussels Sprouts

SERVES 4

Per Serving

Calories	136
Fat	3g
Sodium	320mg
Carbohydrates	24g
Fiber	6g
Sugar	15g
Protein	3g

STORING BUTTERNUT SQUASH

Butternut squash can be stored in a cool, dark place, where it can last for two or three months. Cut and peeled squash can be stored in the refrigerator for up to a week.

The key to getting great-tasting Brussels sprouts is to roast them at a high temperature with something sweet—in this case, butternut squash and maple syrup.

1 large butternut squash, peeled, seeded, and diced (about 4 cups)

1 pound Brussels sprouts, trimmed and halved

1 tablespoon extra-virgin olive oil

2 tablespoons maple syrup

½ teaspoon dried thyme

½ teaspoon salt

¼ teaspoon ground black pepper

1 Preheat oven to 450°F.
2 Combine all ingredients in a large bowl and toss to combine.
3 Spread mixture in a single layer on a large ungreased baking sheet. Bake, stirring once, for 25 minutes or until vegetables are tender. Serve.

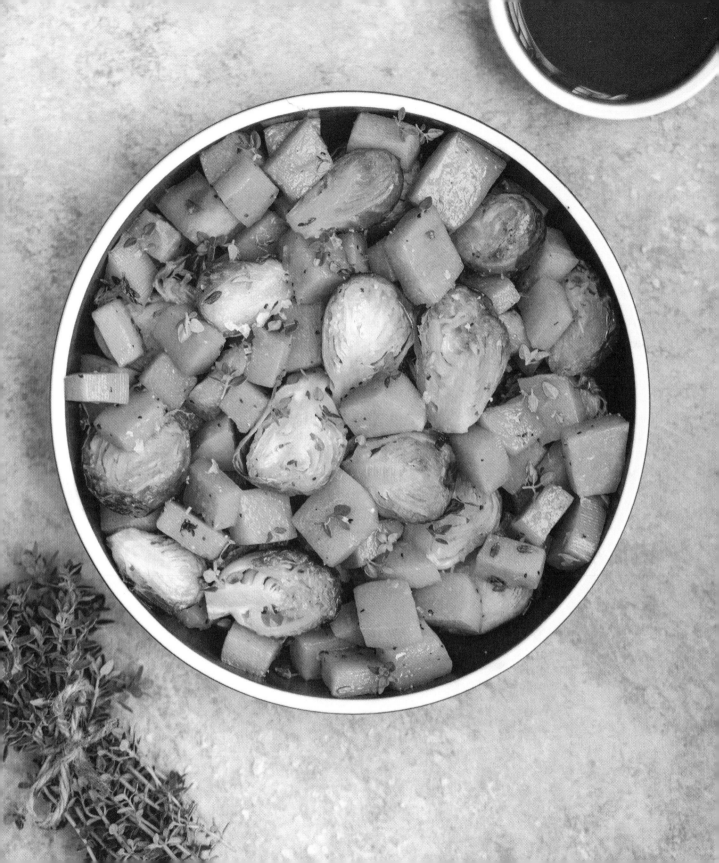

Collard Greens, Potatoes, and White Beans

SERVES 4

Per Serving

Calories	333
Fat	8g
Sodium	252mg
Carbohydrates	52g
Fiber	15g
Sugar	7g
Protein	13g

SOAKING COLLARDS

Collard greens can be pretty dirty, covered in dirt and grime from the fields. Before cooking, soak them in water and vinegar for at least 30 minutes and swish every now and then to loosen dirt. Drain and rinse well, and you're ready to cook delicious and healthy greens!

Closely related to cabbage and kale, collard greens are a great source of vitamin K, which is essential for healthy bones.

1 pound collard greens

1 tablespoon apple cider vinegar

2 tablespoons extra-virgin olive oil

1 medium yellow onion, peeled and diced

3 medium Yukon Gold potatoes, peeled and chopped

1 tablespoon minced fresh oregano

1 (14.5-ounce) can diced tomatoes

1 (15-ounce) can white beans, drained and rinsed

¼ cup water

1 Slice the rib from the center of each collard leaf and discard. Chop leaves into small pieces. Place in a large bowl and cover with cold water; stir in vinegar. Set aside for 30 minutes, then drain and rinse.

2 Heat oil in a large stockpot or Dutch oven over medium heat. Sauté onion until softened, 3–4 minutes. Add collards and cook about 3 minutes until wilted.

3 Add potatoes, oregano, tomatoes, beans, and water. Bring to a boil over high heat. Reduce heat to low, cover, and simmer for 30 minutes or until potatoes are fork-tender. Serve.

Ratatouille

A bright and chunky summer stew that originated in the South of France, ratatouille is known for its soft-cooked vegetables and savory flavor. This dish is a great way to use up vegetables from your summer garden.

1 small eggplant, trimmed and roughly chopped

1 small zucchini squash, trimmed and roughly chopped

1 small yellow squash, trimmed and roughly chopped

1 medium leek, dark green leaves removed and white part roughly chopped

1 large plum tomato, diced

1 small shallot, peeled and minced

2 cloves garlic, peeled and minced

2 sprigs marjoram, stemmed and finely chopped

¼ cup chopped Kalamata olives

½ teaspoon olive oil

1 cup low-sodium vegetable stock

½ teaspoon ground black pepper

1 Place all ingredients in a large saucepan or Dutch oven.

2 Bring to a boil over high heat, then reduce heat to low and simmer for 1½ hours.

3 Serve warm or at room temperature.

SERVES 6

Per Serving

Calories	87
Fat	5g
Sodium	272mg
Carbohydrates	9g
Fiber	3g
Sugar	6g
Protein	2g

Cauliflower Polenta

SERVES 6

Per Serving

Calories	175
Fat	10g
Sodium	382mg
Carbohydrates	14g
Fiber	3g
Sugar	3g
Protein	7g

POLENTA POWER

Polenta is a dish made from boiled cornmeal. It is a great gluten-free alternative as long as wheat flour is not used in its preparation. Polenta is so versatile that it can be served as a meal or as a dessert. Just boil, bake, fry, grill, or microwave polenta at any time of day for a delicious grain alternative to wheat.

Polenta is made from ground corn, and once cooked, it's the perfect bed for sauces and roasted vegetables. Don't confuse polenta with regular cornmeal, which is much more finely ground and is used for baking.

1 medium head cauliflower, stem removed and quartered

4 cups vegetable broth

½ cup yellow corn polenta

½ teaspoon salt

½ cup shredded Cheddar cheese

2 tablespoons butter

1 Coarsely grate the cauliflower and place in a medium saucepan. Add broth, polenta, and salt. Bring to a boil over high heat.

2 Cover and reduce heat to low. Cook, stirring occasionally, until soft and thickened, 20–25 minutes.

3 Remove from heat and stir in cheese and butter. Serve hot.

Irish Colcannon

Colcannon is an authentic Irish dish of mashed potatoes mixed with cabbage or kale and is a St. Patrick's Day favorite.

2 large russet potatoes, peeled and diced

2 tablespoons butter

⅓ cup whole milk

3 tablespoons heavy cream

1 tablespoon olive oil

3 cups trimmed and chopped kale

1 clove garlic, peeled and minced

¼ cup chopped fresh parsley

3 scallions, trimmed and thinly sliced

½ teaspoon salt

¼ teaspoon ground black pepper

SERVES 4	
Per Serving	
Calories	189
Fat	13g
Sodium	304mg
Carbohydrates	15g
Fiber	2g
Sugar	2g
Protein	3g

1 Place potatoes in a large saucepan or Dutch oven. Cover with hot water. Bring to a boil over medium-high heat and cook until fork-tender, about 10 minutes. Drain potatoes and place in a large bowl.

2 Add butter, milk, and cream and beat with an electric mixer until smooth and creamy, 1–2 minutes.

3 Heat oil in the same pan over medium heat. Add kale and garlic and cook, stirring occasionally, until kale has wilted, 3–4 minutes. Add kale mixture to whipped potatoes and stir to combine.

4 Stir in parsley, scallions, salt, and pepper. Serve hot.

Vegan Creamed Spinach

To boost nutrition and anti-inflammation effects, try to eat two cups of dark, leafy greens per day. This spinach side dish makes that goal easy and delicious.

2 tablespoons vegan butter

1 medium yellow onion, peeled and diced

2 cloves garlic, peeled and minced

2 tablespoons all-purpose flour

2 cups almond milk

2 tablespoons nutritional yeast

16 ounces frozen spinach, thawed and drained

1 Melt vegan butter in a large skillet over medium heat. Sauté onion until softened, 3–4 minutes. Add garlic and sauté for 30 seconds. Sprinkle with flour and stir.

2 Add almond milk slowly, stirring often, until thickened, 3–4 minutes. Stir in yeast and spinach. Serve hot.

Mixed Potato Pancakes

Sweet potato, an excellent source of vitamin A, makes a great addition to the classic potato pancake. Try topping these pancakes with fried eggs for breakfast.

1 large sweet potato, peeled and shredded

1 large baking potato, peeled and shredded

1 tablespoon olive oil

1 In a medium bowl, combine potatoes. Form into small patties, about 2½" in diameter.

2 Heat oil in a large skillet over medium-high heat. Place patties in the skillet. Cook, turning once, until browned on each side, about 3 minutes per side. Serve immediately.

SERVES 6

Per Serving

Calories	89
Fat	2g
Sodium	5mg
Carbohydrates	16g
Fiber	2g
Sugar	0g
Protein	2g

Potato Gnocchi with Tomato Basil Sauce

SERVES 6

Per Serving

Calories	235
Fat	5g
Sodium	526mg
Carbohydrates	38g
Fiber	5g
Sugar	8g
Protein	10g

GROWING FRESH BASIL

Always have a supply of fresh basil by keeping a plant growing year-round. In the spring and fall months, put a pot with a fresh basil plant outside on your patio. During the cold winter months and hot summer, move it indoors by a sunny window. Wait until the soil is dry before watering.

To obtain optimum flavor, toss the cooked gnocchi in a sauté pan with the sauce for 1–2 minutes.

1 medium potato, peeled
¾ cup whole-wheat flour
¾ cup all-purpose flour
2 large egg whites
¼ cup low-sodium vegetable stock
⅛ teaspoon plus 1 tablespoon salt, divided
1 teaspoon olive oil
2 cups Fresh Tomato Sauce (see recipe in Chapter 6)
¼ cup grated Romano cheese
3 large basil leaves, thinly sliced
½ teaspoon ground black pepper

1. Place potato in a small saucepan and cover with water. Boil over medium-high heat until tender when pierced with a fork, about 20 minutes.
2. Using a stand mixer fitted with a dough hook, mix together potato, flours, egg whites, stock, ⅛ teaspoon salt, and oil for about 1 minute at low speed until ingredients are thoroughly incorporated. (This kneading can also be done by hand.) Set aside to rest for 1 hour.
3. Fill a large pot with water and add remaining 1 tablespoon salt. Bring to a boil over high heat. Heat Fresh Tomato Sauce in a medium saucepan over medium heat for 10 minutes. Keep warm over very low heat.
4. On a floured work surface, roll dough using both hands to form a long ½"-thick "rope," then slice into 1"-long pieces. Place pieces in boiling water and cook for 3–5 minutes until the gnocchi float to the surface. Drain and transfer to a large bowl or serving platter.
5. Ladle sauce over gnocchi, then sprinkle with cheese, basil, and pepper. Serve immediately.

Roasted Kale Chips

Kale contains chlorophyll, a plant pigment that helps prevent the absorption of heterocyclic amines—carcinogens created when animal proteins are cooked at a high temperature. The next time you eat a chargrilled steak or chicken, pair it with a side of green vegetables to reduce the impact.

6 cups trimmed and chopped kale

1 tablespoon extra-virgin olive oil

1 teaspoon garlic powder

½ teaspoon flaky salt

1 Preheat oven to 375°F.
2 Place kale in a large bowl; toss with oil and garlic powder. Transfer kale to a large ungreased baking sheet.
3 Roast for 5 minutes; turn kale over and roast another 7–10 minutes until kale turns brown and becomes paper-thin and brittle.
4 Remove from oven and sprinkle with salt. Serve immediately.

SERVES 2

Per Serving

Calories	91
Fat	8g
Sodium	524mg
Carbohydrates	3g
Fiber	3g
Sugar	1g
Protein	2g

CHAPTER 6

Salads, Dressings, and Sauces

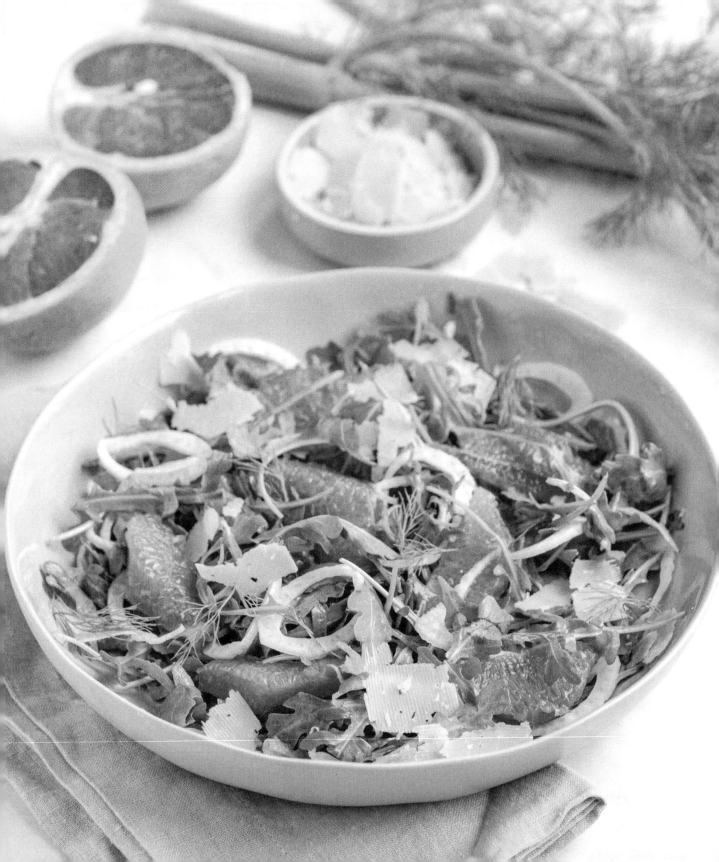

Grapefruit Fennel Salad

Fennel is sweet, crunchy, and refreshing. Baby arugula is tender and slightly peppery. When you add tart grapefruit into the mix, you get a citrusy taste that binds it all together.

1 medium fennel bulb

2 large grapefruit

¼ cup extra-virgin olive oil

3 tablespoons lemon juice

1 teaspoon honey

½ teaspoon table salt

¼ teaspoon ground black pepper

5 ounces baby arugula

¼ cup shaved Parmesan cheese

½ teaspoon flaky sea salt

1 Cut green stems from fennel bulb and discard. Thinly slice with a mandoline.
2 Using a sharp knife, remove the peel and membranes from grapefruit and slice into pieces.
3 In a large bowl, whisk together oil, lemon juice, honey, table salt, and pepper. Add fennel, grapefruit, arugula, and Parmesan. Toss to combine. Sprinkle with flaky sea salt before serving.

SERVES 4

Per Serving

Calories	246
Fat	16g
Sodium	390mg
Carbohydrates	23g
Fiber	4g
Sugar	14g
Protein	3g

GRAPEFRUIT

Some find grapefruit to be a bit too sour. To reduce the bitterness, sprinkle the segments with a small amount of sugar.

Apple, Ginger, and Carrot Salad

SERVES 4

Per Serving

Calories	311
Fat	21g
Sodium	31mg
Carbohydrates	28g
Fiber	5g
Sugar	20g
Protein	3g

For a sweet salad, use red apples, but green Granny Smith apples will balance out the carrots and cranberries.

2 large apples, peeled, cored, and chopped

2 teaspoons lemon juice

2 large carrots, peeled and grated

¼ cup dried cranberries

12 walnut halves

1 (2") piece fresh ginger

¼ cup extra-virgin olive oil

¼ cup white balsamic vinegar

1 teaspoon ume plum vinegar

5 ounces baby arugula or spinach

1 Place apples in a medium bowl and sprinkle with lemon juice. Toss to coat. Add carrots, cranberries, and walnuts.

2 Using a fine grater, grate ginger and squeeze or press to extract 1 teaspoon juice into a small bowl.

3 Add oil, balsamic vinegar, and plum vinegar to the small bowl and whisk to combine. Pour dressing over apple mixture and toss to combine.

4 Place arugula on a large platter. Top with apple salad and serve immediately.

Sunshine Salad

Sunflower seeds are an excellent source of selenium and vitamin E, nutrients that help fight off chronic disease. They are also rich in heart-healthy fats.

6 ounces low-fat plain Greek yogurt

2 tablespoons sour cream

2 tablespoons mayonnaise

1 tablespoon grated lemon zest

¼ teaspoon crushed red pepper flakes

⅛ teaspoon seasoned salt

6 cups baby spinach

1 large cucumber, peeled, seeded, and sliced into half-moons

1 cup canned mandarin oranges, drained

1 cup halved cherry tomatoes

½ cup roasted shelled sunflower seeds, divided

1 In a small bowl, combine yogurt, sour cream, mayonnaise, lemon zest, crushed red pepper flakes, and seasoned salt; stir until well blended.

2 In a large bowl, combine spinach, cucumber, oranges, cherry tomatoes, and ¼ cup sunflower seeds. Add dressing and toss to coat.

3 To serve, transfer salad to a chilled bowl and top with the remaining ¼ cup sunflower seeds.

SERVES 4

Per Serving

Calories	196
Fat	10g
Sodium	173mg
Carbohydrates	20g
Fiber	4g
Sugar	13g
Protein	7g

GREEK YOGURT

Greek yogurt has a thicker consistency, more protein, and less sugar than regular yogurt. It's made by removing the whey—the liquid that remains after milk has been curdled and strained—in the yogurt-making process.

Tomato Salad with Basil Pine Nut Dressing

SERVES 6

Per Serving

Calories	193
Fat	17g
Sodium	268mg
Carbohydrates	8g
Fiber	1g
Sugar	2g
Protein	2g

Pine nuts, found in pinecones, have a soft, buttery texture. They're high in vitamin K, phosphorus, and magnesium, all essential for healthy bones.

1 large Vidalia onion, peeled and thinly sliced

4 large ripe tomatoes, cut into large wedges

3 tablespoons extra-virgin olive oil

⅓ cup pine nuts

6 cloves roasted garlic

½ bunch fresh basil, stemmed and thinly sliced

½ teaspoon ground black pepper

¼ cup sliced Kalamata olives

1 Combine onion and tomatoes in a large bowl and drizzle with oil.
2 Place pine nuts in a small ungreased skillet over medium heat and toast, stirring, until light brown, 1–2 minutes.
3 In a food processor or blender, process garlic to form a paste, then add pine nuts, basil, and pepper. Pulse two or three times to combine.
4 Dollop garlic mixture over tomatoes and onion. Top with olive slices and serve immediately.

Quinoa, Raisin, and Bok Choy Salad

Crunchy and delicious, baby bok choy is a member of the cruciferous vegetable family. It's full of healthy antioxidants.

1 cup quinoa, rinsed and drained

2 cups vegetable broth

4 small baby bok choy, trimmed and thinly sliced

1 large English cucumber, sliced into half-moons

3 medium radishes, trimmed and thinly sliced

½ cup golden raisins

1 recipe Miso Carrot Salad Dressing (see recipe in this chapter)

SERVES 4	
Per Serving	
Calories	258
Fat	5g
Sodium	111mg
Carbohydrates	46g
Fiber	4g
Sugar	16g
Protein	7g

1 Place quinoa and broth in a medium saucepan. Bring to a boil over high heat. Reduce heat to medium-low, cover, and simmer for 15 minutes. Remove from heat and spread out onto a baking sheet to cool.

2 Transfer cooled quinoa to a large bowl. Add bok choy, cucumber, radishes, and raisins. Pour Miso Carrot Salad Dressing over the mixture and toss to combine. Serve immediately.

Vegan Niçoise Salad Bowls

SERVES 4

Per Serving

Calories	596
Fat	21g
Sodium	423mg
Carbohydrates	80g
Fiber	19g
Sugar	14g
Protein	22g

ARTICHOKES: CANNED OR FRESH?

Fresh artichokes can be hard to find and difficult to prepare. Canned or jarred artichokes are available year-round and come packed in brine or a marinade, which can add a delicious Italian flavor to dishes.

Niçoise *means "in the style of Nice, France." This region is known for its olives, tomatoes, and beans.*

¼ cup tahini

3 tablespoons water

3 tablespoons lemon juice

1 tablespoon seasoned rice vinegar

1 tablespoon extra-virgin olive oil

1 teaspoon low-sodium soy sauce

2 cloves garlic, peeled and minced

½ small shallot, peeled and minced

¼ teaspoon salt

⅛ teaspoon ground black pepper

1 pound baby red potatoes, halved

8 ounces fresh green beans, trimmed

2 heads butter lettuce, torn into bite-sized pieces

1 (15-ounce) can artichoke hearts in brine, drained and chopped

1 (15-ounce) can chickpeas, drained and rinsed

1 pint cherry tomatoes, halved

½ small red onion, peeled and thinly sliced

¼ cup Kalamata olives

1. In a small bowl, whisk together tahini, water, lemon juice, vinegar, oil, soy sauce, garlic, shallot, salt, and pepper. Set aside.
2. Place potatoes in a steamer basket in a large pot. Add water to just below the basket and bring to a boil over high heat. Cover and steam potatoes for 10–12 minutes until tender. Transfer potatoes to a large bowl and let cool.
3. Return the steamer basket to the pot; add green beans and more water. Cover and steam green beans over high heat for 4–5 minutes until crisp-tender. Add beans to the bowl with potatoes.
4. Divide lettuce among four bowls or salad plates.
5. Arrange potatoes, green beans, artichokes, chickpeas, tomatoes, onion, and olives over lettuce. Drizzle with dressing. Serve immediately.

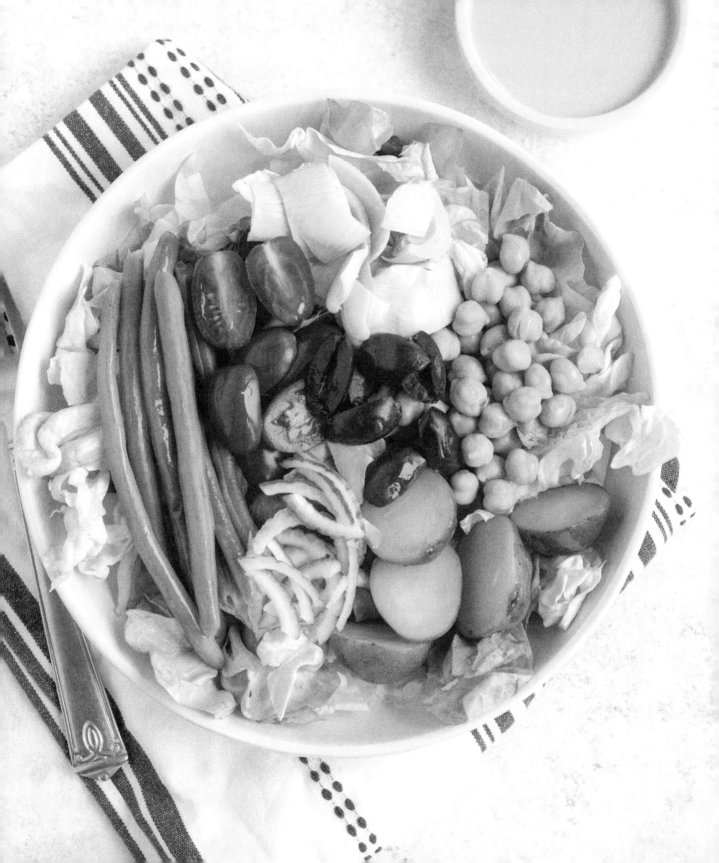

Green Lentil Salad

SERVES 4

Per Serving

Calories	275
Fat	15g
Sodium	315mg
Carbohydrates	20g
Fiber	1g
Sugar	2g
Protein	15g

IRON POWER

Lentils are one of the best vegetable sources of iron. They are ideal for vegetarians and help prevent iron deficiency anemia. They are also an excellent source of protein and fiber, which allows meals to keep you satisfied for hours.

Green lentils are smaller and plumper than other lentils, which is why they're sometimes called "the caviar of lentils." This dish is seasoned with ground coriander, which is made from dried cilantro seeds. Coriander has a milder and sweeter flavor than fresh cilantro.

1 cup dried French green lentils

5 cups water

1 bay leaf

2 tablespoons light olive oil

1 large carrot, peeled and finely chopped

1 stalk celery, trimmed and finely chopped

2 tablespoons minced shallot

1 teaspoon minced garlic

2 tablespoons extra-virgin olive oil

¼ cup lemon juice

1 teaspoon grated lemon zest

1 tablespoon chopped fresh thyme

1 tablespoon chopped fresh parsley

¼ teaspoon ground coriander

½ teaspoon salt

½ teaspoon ground black pepper

1 Place lentils, water, and bay leaf in a large saucepan. Bring to a boil over high heat. Reduce heat to medium-low and simmer for 20 minutes. Drain lentils, remove and discard bay leaf, and transfer lentils to a large bowl. Set aside.

2 Heat light olive oil in a medium skillet over medium heat. Sauté carrot, celery, and shallots until tender, about 5 minutes. Add carrot mixture to lentils.

3 Add garlic, extra-virgin olive oil, lemon juice, lemon zest, thyme, parsley, coriander, salt, and pepper to the lentils. Toss to combine.

4 Refrigerate for at least 2 hours. Serve chilled or at room temperature.

Potato and Chickpea Curry Salad

Curry powder is a mix of many different spices, usually coriander, cumin, turmeric, ginger, dried mustard, cinnamon, and cardamom. These spices are all known for their antioxidant properties. You can buy premade curry powder or make your own mix from many recipes found online.

1 teaspoon olive oil

1 large yellow onion, peeled and sliced

1 cup dried chickpeas

1½ tablespoons curry powder

3 cloves garlic, peeled and minced

1 bay leaf

4 cups low-sodium vegetable stock

2 large baked potatoes, cubed

3 stalks celery, trimmed and diced

1 pint cherry tomatoes, halved

¾ teaspoon salt

½ teaspoon ground black pepper

SERVES 6	
Per Serving	
Calories	131
Fat	2g
Sodium	320mg
Carbohydrates	23g
Fiber	4g
Sugar	6g
Protein	5g

1   Heat oil in a large stockpot or Dutch oven over medium-high heat. Sauté onion until soft, about 5 minutes. Add chickpeas, curry, garlic, bay leaf, and stock. Bring to a boil, then reduce heat to low. Simmer for 2 hours.

2   Drain chickpeas, remove and discard bay leaf, and transfer chickpea mixture to a large bowl. Set aside to cool for 30 minutes.

3   Add potatoes, celery, and tomatoes to chickpeas and stir gently to combine. Season with salt and pepper. Serve at room temperature or refrigerate for up to 5 days.

Three-Bean Salad

MARJORAM

Marjoram is an herb that is similar to oregano, but it's sweeter in flavor. If you can't find fresh marjoram, substitute equal parts fresh oregano.

Feel free to switch up the beans and vinegar in this recipe—yellow wax beans and white vinegar make a great variation.

1 cup fresh trimmed green beans

1 large red onion, peeled and thinly sliced

3 sprigs marjoram, stemmed and chopped

¼ cup chopped Kalamata olives

½ cup cooked red kidney beans

½ cup cooked chickpeas or cannellini beans

2 tablespoons extra-virgin olive oil

½ cup balsamic vinegar

½ teaspoon ground black pepper

1 Bring 1" water to a boil in a medium saucepan over medium-high heat. Place a steamer insert in the pan and add green beans. Cover and steam for 3–5 minutes until just tender. Transfer beans to a colander and rinse in cold water. Drain thoroughly and transfer to a large bowl.

2 Add remaining ingredients and toss to combine. Serve at room temperature or refrigerate for at least 2 hours.

Coleslaw

Fresh homemade coleslaw is a delicious way to get more cabbage into your diet. Coleslaw keeps for days in the refrigerator. In fact, the flavor tends to get better as time goes on!

3 cups shredded green cabbage

¼ cup shredded carrot

¼ cup sliced scallions

¼ cup canola oil

1 teaspoon sesame oil

2 tablespoons rice vinegar

1 tablespoon sesame seeds

½ teaspoon salt

½ teaspoon ground black pepper

Combine all ingredients in a large bowl. Cover and refrigerate for at least 1 hour before serving.

SERVES 4

Per Serving

Calories	166
Fat	16g
Sodium	309mg
Carbohydrates	5g
Fiber	2g
Sugar	2g
Protein	1g

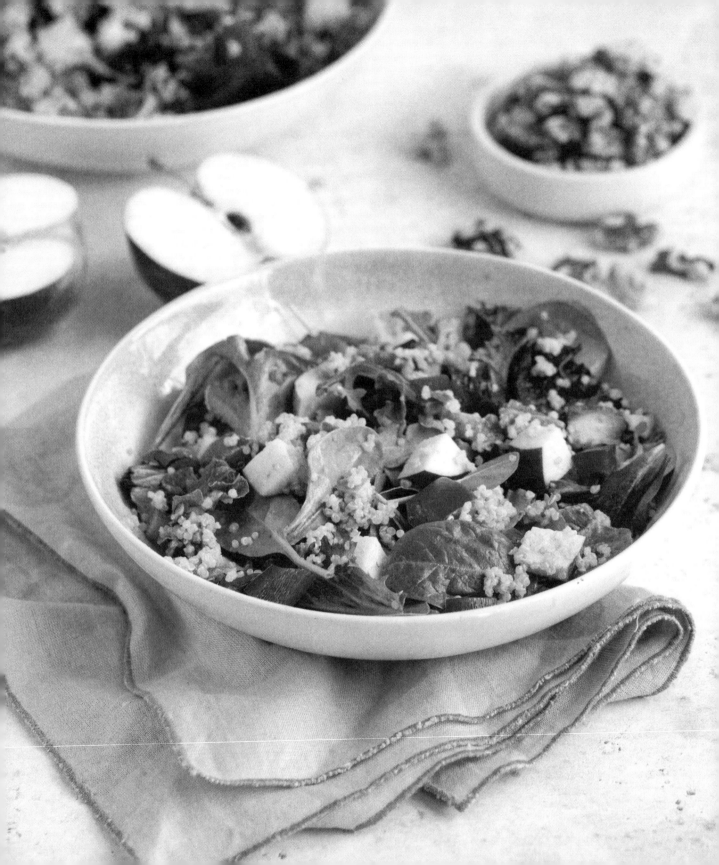

Quinoa Apple Salad

Quinoa is rich in both fiber and protein, and has a fluffy texture that's similar to rice. Be sure to rinse it in a strainer under cool water before cooking to remove bitterness.

1 cup plus 2 tablespoons water, divided

⅓ cup quinoa, rinsed and drained

¼ cup olive oil

2 tablespoons apple cider vinegar

2 cloves garlic, peeled

1 tablespoon agave syrup

2 large pitted dates

⅛ teaspoon ground cinnamon

5 ounces spring greens

1 large red bell pepper, seeded and chopped

2 medium apples, cored and chopped

1 cup chopped walnuts

1 Combine 1 cup water and quinoa in a medium saucepan over high heat. Cover and bring to a boil. Reduce heat to low and simmer on low heat until all water is absorbed, 10–15 minutes. Set aside to cool for 15 minutes.

2 In a blender or food processor, purée oil, vinegar, garlic, agave, dates, and cinnamon. Slowly add remaining 2 tablespoons water until mixture is thinned to a salad dressing consistency.

3 Pour dressing in the bottom of a large salad bowl. Add greens, pepper, apples, quinoa, and walnuts. Toss well. Serve immediately.

SERVES 8

Per Serving

Calories	240
Fat	16g
Sodium	13mg
Carbohydrates	20g
Fiber	4g
Sugar	12g
Protein	4g

AGAVE SYRUP

Agave syrup is a sweetener made from the sap of the blue agave plant. Blue agave is considered to be the finest in the world. High-quality tequilas are also produced from the blue agave plant.

Broccoli Raisin Slaw

SERVES 4

Per Serving

Calories	177
Fat	12g
Sodium	343mg
Carbohydrates	11g
Fiber	3g
Sugar	8g
Protein	6g

Golden raisins are made from white grapes and tend to be fruitier tasting, plumper, and softer than their brown counterparts.

3 cups blanched broccoli florets

¼ cup shredded carrot

2 tablespoons mayonnaise

1 teaspoon Dijon mustard

1 tablespoon red wine vinegar

1 tablespoon minced shallot

¼ cup golden raisins

½ cup toasted sliced almonds

½ teaspoon salt

½ teaspoon ground black pepper

Combine all ingredients in a large bowl. Cover and refrigerate for at least 1 hour before serving.

Quinoa Black Bean Salad

The longer a grain salad marinates, the better the flavors are absorbed by the ingredients. Make this salad the night before and take some to work for lunch the next day.

1 cup quinoa, rinsed and drained

2 cups water

1 teaspoon salt, divided

1 medium carrot, peeled and grated

2 scallions, trimmed and sliced

⅓ cup pumpkin seeds

½ cup chopped fresh parsley

1 (14-ounce) can black beans, drained and rinsed

3 tablespoons lemon juice

1 clove garlic, peeled and minced

2 tablespoons apple cider vinegar

3 tablespoons extra-virgin olive oil

1 In a medium saucepan, combine quinoa, water, and ½ teaspoon salt. Cover, bring to a boil over high heat, reduce heat to low, and simmer until all water is absorbed, about 20 minutes.

2 Spoon quinoa into a large bowl and set aside to cool for at least 20 minutes.

3 When quinoa is cool, add carrot, scallions, pumpkin seeds, parsley, and black beans; mix well.

4 In a small bowl, whisk together lemon juice, garlic, vinegar, oil, and remaining ½ teaspoon salt. Pour dressing over quinoa mixture and toss to mix.

5 Set aside for 15 minutes before serving.

SERVES 8

Per Serving

Calories	241
Fat	11g
Sodium	302mg
Carbohydrates	24g
Fiber	6g
Sugar	0g
Protein	12g

TOASTING PUMPKIN SEEDS

Raw pumpkin seeds can be toasted in a dry skillet over medium-low heat. Keep them moving around by shaking the pan from time to time or stirring them with a wooden spoon. You'll know they are done when they've stopped popping and turned a golden brown.

Asian Fusion Salad

SERVES 4

Per Serving

Calories	192
Fat	12g
Sodium	456mg
Carbohydrates	17g
Fiber	1g
Sugar	5g
Protein	4g

Watercress is a leafy green vegetable with a mild peppery flavor. If you can't find it in your grocery store, substitute baby arugula.

3 tablespoons light coconut milk

3 tablespoons Thai chili sauce

2 tablespoons low-sodium soy sauce

1 tablespoon olive oil

2 cups baby spinach

1 bunch watercress, trimmed

1 (8-ounce) can sliced water chestnuts

8 sesame-flavored rice crackers, crumbled

½ cup chopped cashews

1 In a small bowl, combine coconut milk, chili sauce, soy sauce, and oil; mix well and set aside.

2 Combine spinach, watercress, and water chestnuts in a large bowl, add dressing, and toss until leaves are well coated. Sprinkle with crumbled crackers and cashews, toss again, and serve.

Sweet and Sour Cucumber Relish

Use this relish to top grilled chicken or turkey sausages, or just eat it as a crunchy side dish with any meal.

1 large English cucumber, peeled and diced

2 teaspoons grated lime zest

2 tablespoons lime juice

1 teaspoon honey

1 teaspoon white vinegar

Combine all ingredients in a medium bowl. Cover and refrigerate for at least 1 hour before serving.

SERVES 8

Per Serving

Calories	8
Fat	0g
Sodium	1mg
Carbohydrates	2g
Fiber	0g
Sugar	1g
Protein	0g

DIFFERENCE IN CUCUMBERS

The main difference between English cucumbers and regular cucumbers is that English cucumbers have thinner skin and much smaller (almost nonexistant) seeds. They also taste a bit sweeter. To substitute regular cucumbers for English, simply remove the seeds.

Jalapeño Corn Salad Dressing

SERVES 4

Per Serving

Calories	111
Fat	8g
Sodium	407mg
Carbohydrates	6g
Fiber	1g
Sugar	2g
Protein	3g

USING FRESH CORN

Fresh corn tastes best in the summertime, when the kernels are bright yellow. When you can find fresh summer corn, use it in recipes by cooking it first. Preheat oven to 400°F and trim the ends of the husks. Place corncobs (in husks) directly on oven racks and bake for 30 minutes. Let cool before shucking, then slice off kernels with a sharp knife to add to a variety of recipes. Or just eat the corn right off the cob!

Add this creamy dressing to potato or pasta salad for a sweet and spicy kick.

10 ounces frozen corn kernels, thawed

1 medium jalapeño pepper, seeded and minced

½ cup water

2 tablespoons extra-virgin olive oil

1 tablespoon chopped fresh dill

1 tablespoon sliced scallions

1 teaspoon Dijon mustard

2 cloves garlic, peeled and minced

½ teaspoon salt

½ teaspoon ground black pepper

1 Place corn, jalapeño, and water in a blender. Blend until smooth.

2 Press mixture through a mesh strainer into a medium bowl and discard the solids. Whisk in oil, dill, scallions, mustard, garlic, salt, and black pepper. Serve immediately or refrigerate for up to 5 days.

Citrus Vinaigrette

Oranges, lemons, and other citrus fruits contain flavonoids, plant compounds that may protect against esophageal, stomach, breast, and pancreatic cancers.

2½ tablespoons lemon juice

2½ tablespoons orange juice

1 teaspoon honey

½ tablespoon grated lemon zest

½ tablespoon grated orange zest

½ teaspoon salt

½ teaspoon ground black pepper

⅔ cup extra-virgin olive oil

SERVES 8	
Per Serving	
Calories	178
Fat	19g
Sodium	145mg
Carbohydrates	2g
Fiber	0g
Sugar	1g
Protein	0g

Combine lemon and orange juices, honey, zests, salt, and pepper in a container or jar with cover and shake vigorously to combine. Add oil and shake until emulsified. Alternatively, combine all ingredients in a blender or food processor and process until creamy. Use immediately or refrigerate overnight. Bring to room temperature before using.

Miso Carrot Salad Dressing

SERVES 4

Per Serving

Calories	193
Fat	14g
Sodium	649mg
Carbohydrates	15g
Fiber	2g
Sugar	8g
Protein	2g

STORING OIL-BASED DRESSINGS

If you have extra salad dressing that you store in the refrigerator, it will likely separate. To recombine before using, let the dressing sit out at room temperature for about 30 minutes, then shake well.

This smooth bright orange-yellow dressing contains ginger, which is loaded with antioxidants that help prevent damage to your body's DNA. Carrots are high in vitamin A, which promotes healthy vision and healthy aging.

¼ cup grapeseed oil

¼ cup apple cider vinegar

3 tablespoons white miso

1 tablespoon maple syrup

2 large carrots, peeled and grated

1 tablespoon minced fresh ginger

½ teaspoon salt

½ teaspoon ground black pepper

Place all ingredients in a blender and purée until smooth. Serve immediately or refrigerate for up to 5 days.

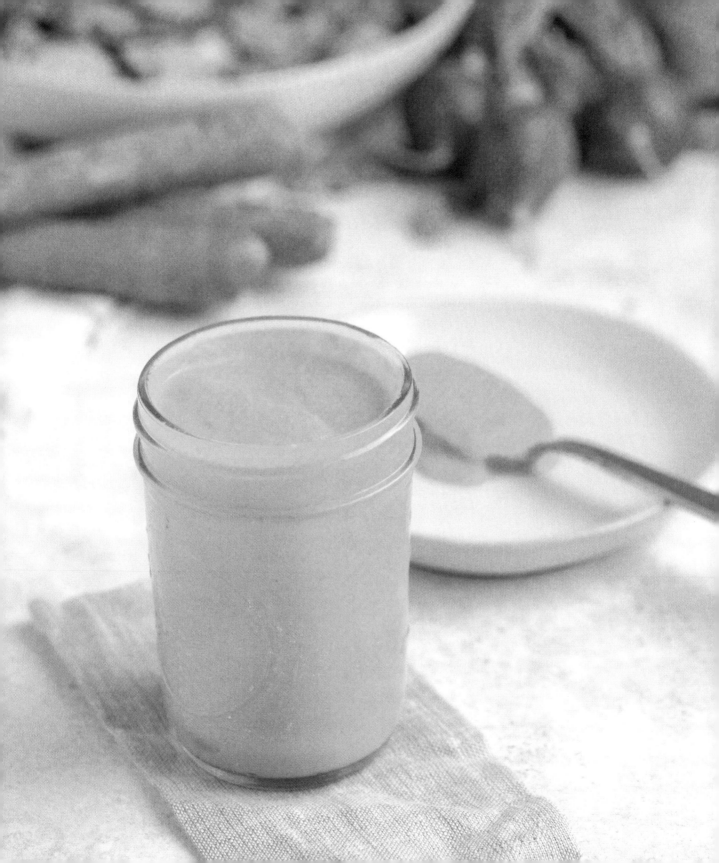

Lemon Poppy Seed Salad Dressing

SERVES 8

Per Serving

Calories	202
Fat	19g
Sodium	77mg
Carbohydrates	8g
Fiber	0g
Sugar	7g
Protein	0g

Poppy seeds provide a tasty crunch to this dressing. The seeds are so tiny that they disperse evenly throughout a salad and add a little crunch to each bite.

¼ cup sugar

¼ cup lemon juice

¼ teaspoon Dijon mustard

¼ teaspoon salt

⅛ teaspoon onion powder

⅔ cup extra-virgin olive oil

½ tablespoon poppy seeds

To a small bowl, add sugar, lemon juice, mustard, salt, and onion powder. Whisk to combine. Add oil in a slow, steady stream, whisking constantly, until mixture is thick and smooth. Add poppy seeds, and whisk further to combine. Serve immediately or refrigerate for up to 5 days.

Creamy Oregano Dijon Salad Dressing

SERVES 4

Per Serving

Calories	107
Fat	10g
Sodium	761mg
Carbohydrates	4g
Fiber	0g
Sugar	3g
Protein	0g

Dried oregano is loaded with the antioxidants thymol and limonene, which can help fight free radical damage.

4 cloves garlic, peeled and minced

¼ cup mayonnaise or vegan mayonnaise

1 tablespoon white wine vinegar

1 tablespoon Dijon mustard

1 tablespoon honey or maple syrup

1 teaspoon dried oregano

1 teaspoon salt

½ teaspoon ground black pepper

Place all ingredients in a small bowl and whisk until combined. Serve immediately or refrigerate for up to 5 days.

Savory Marinade for Meats, Fish, and Poultry

This is a basic flavorful marinade great for chicken, beef, or fish. It also works well on grilled vegetables.

2/3 cup red wine vinegar

1/3 cup vegetable oil

2 tablespoons Dijon mustard

2 tablespoons Worcestershire sauce

2 cloves garlic, peeled and minced

1 tablespoon chopped fresh parsley

1/4 teaspoon paprika

1/8 teaspoon ground black pepper

1 bay leaf, broken into pieces

Combine all ingredients in a glass bowl and mix well. Use immediately or refrigerate for up to 5 days.

SERVES 6	
Per Serving	
Calories	124
Fat	13g
Sodium	191mg
Carbohydrates	1g
Fiber	0g
Sugar	1g
Protein	0g

Tropical Marinade for Chicken

Reserve about 1/2 cup of the marinade in a separate, clean bowl before adding the rest to the chicken. Brush chicken with reserved marinade just before serving.

2/3 cup pineapple juice

1/3 cup vegetable oil

2 cloves garlic, peeled and minced

1/4 teaspoon paprika

1 teaspoon ground cumin

1/4 teaspoon ground ginger

1/8 teaspoon ground nutmeg

1/8 teaspoon ground allspice

1/8 teaspoon ground black pepper

Combine all ingredients in a medium bowl and mix well. Use immediately or refrigerate for up to 5 days.

SERVES 12	
Per Serving	
Calories	62
Fat	6g
Sodium	0mg
Carbohydrates	2g
Fiber	0g
Sugar	1g
Protein	0g

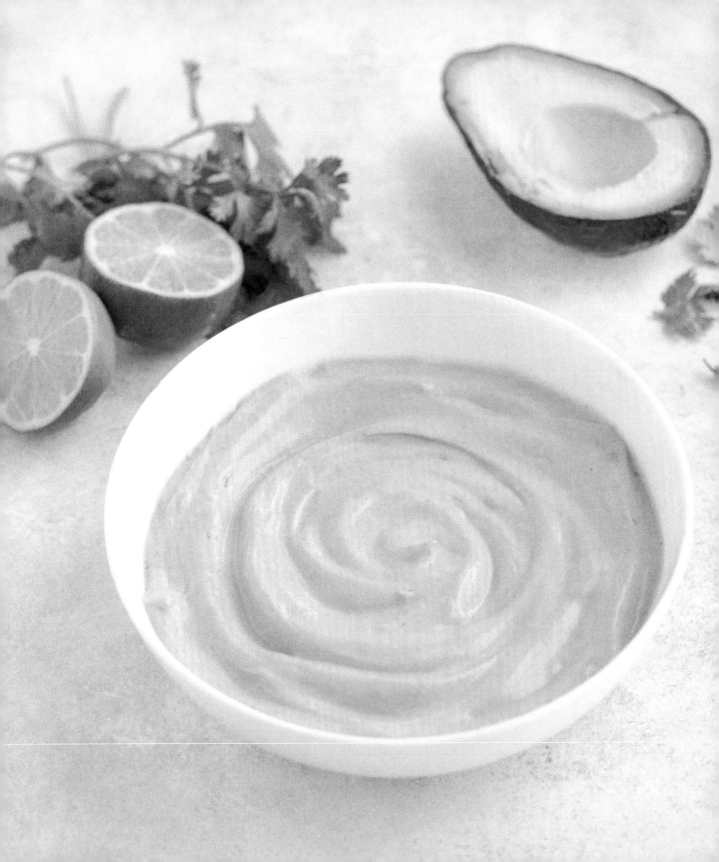

Vegan Avocado Crema

Rich in heart-healthy fats, avocados are creamy and filling. Use this avocado crema on tacos, enchiladas, sandwiches, or savory oatmeal bowls.

1 large ripe avocado, peeled and pitted

1 tablespoon lime juice

¼ cup vegan sour cream

¼ cup loosely packed cilantro leaves

¼ cup water

¼ teaspoon salt

Add all ingredients to a blender and purée until smooth. Serve immediately.

SERVES 4

Per Serving

Calories	115
Fat	11g
Sodium	188mg
Carbohydrates	3g
Fiber	3g
Sugar	0g
Protein	1g

AVOCADOS

Any recipe that includes avocados should be eaten immediately. When sliced or mashed avocados are stored in the refrigerator, they tend to turn brown. You can combat this by squeezing lemon or lime juice over avocados, which will extend the green for a little bit.

Thai Peanut Sauce

SERVES 4

Per Serving

Calories	138
Fat	11g
Sodium	305mg
Carbohydrates	5g
Fiber	1g
Sugar	2g
Protein	5g

TAMARI VS. SOY SAUCE

Tamari and soy sauce are both derived from fermented soybeans, but tamari is made without wheat, which is great for those who need to be gluten-free.

This is a great sauce for freshly made spring rolls or stir-fried tofu. Crushed red pepper flakes add a delicious spicy kick.

2 tablespoons water

¼ cup creamy peanut butter

2 tablespoons tamari

1 teaspoon crushed red pepper flakes

2 teaspoons sesame oil

2 tablespoons chopped unsalted peanuts

1 Place water, peanut butter, tamari, crushed red pepper flakes, and oil in a food processor or blender; process until smooth. Add a little more water if necessary to adjust the consistency.

2 Place sauce in a small serving bowl and garnish with peanuts. Serve immediately or refrigerate for up to 5 days.

Fresh Tomato Sauce

If you find yourself with an excess of summer tomatoes from your garden, use them in this delicious Fresh Tomato Sauce. Packed with fresh herbs and garlic, this tomato sauce goes great on pasta and homemade gnocchi.

1 tablespoon olive oil

2 large yellow onions, peeled and diced

1 medium shallot, peeled and minced

8 cloves garlic, peeled and minced

20 medium plum tomatoes, chopped

½ cup dry red wine

10 large basil leaves, chopped

3 sprigs fresh oregano, stemmed and chopped

¼ bunch fresh parsley, stemmed and chopped

1 teaspoon ground black pepper

2 tablespoons cold unsalted butter

MAKES 2 CUPS	
Per Serving (½ cup)	
Calories	168
Fat	9g
Sodium	18mg
Carbohydrates	16g
Fiber	7g
Sugar	15g
Protein	6g

1 Heat oil in a large stockpot over medium-high heat. Add onions, shallot, and garlic. Sauté lightly for 3 minutes, then add tomatoes. Sauté 3 minutes. Add wine and reduce heat to medium-low. Simmer until slightly thickened, about 10 minutes.

2 Stir in basil, oregano, parsley, and pepper. Remove from heat and add butter. Stir until butter melts. Serve immediately or refrigerate for up to 5 days.

Basil Pine Nut Pesto

SERVES 4	
Per Serving	
Calories	249
Fat	26g
Sodium	291mg
Carbohydrates	2g
Fiber	0g
Sugar	0g
Protein	2g

If you like, stir in a handful of grated Parmesan cheese after you have removed the pesto from the food processor or blender.

½ cup pine nuts

8 cloves garlic, peeled

¼ bunch basil, roughly chopped

¼ cup olive oil

½ teaspoon salt

½ teaspoon ground black pepper

1 Place pine nuts in a blender or food processor and process for 30 seconds. Add garlic and blend until the mixture forms a paste, about 1 minute. Add basil and blend to combine.

2 While the blender is running, drizzle in oil until mixture is smooth, about 1 minute more. Transfer to a small bowl and season with salt and pepper. Serve immediately or refrigerate for up to 5 days.

Walnut Parsley Pesto

SERVES 4	
Per Serving	
Calories	215
Fat	22g
Sodium	291mg
Carbohydrates	2g
Fiber	1g
Sugar	0g
Protein	2g

Walnuts are an excellent source of omega-3 fatty acids, with more than other tree nuts. They're also a good source of protein, fiber, and magnesium, which is essential for muscle and nerve function.

½ cup walnut halves

8 cloves garlic, peeled

1 bunch parsley, roughly chopped

¼ cup olive oil

½ teaspoon salt

½ teaspoon ground black pepper

1 Place walnuts in a blender or food processor and process for 30 seconds. Add garlic and blend until the mixture forms a paste, about 1 minute. Add parsley and blend to combine.

2 While the blender is running, drizzle in oil until mixture is smooth, about 1 minute more. Transfer to a small bowl and season with salt and pepper. Serve immediately or refrigerate for up to 5 days.

Pasta and Grains

Pasta e Ceci

SERVES 4

Per Serving

Calories	508
Fat	19g
Sodium	597mg
Carbohydrates	69g
Fiber	6g
Sugar	3g
Protein	16g

Lagane e ceci, a dish from southeastern Italy, consists of a home-made wide pasta with chickpeas, garlic, and oil. You don't need to make your own pasta to enjoy this comforting dish. Use your favorite flat pasta such as linguine, fettuccine, or egg noodles.

4 tablespoons extra-virgin olive oil, divided

½ teaspoon onion powder

½ teaspoon dried rosemary

2 teaspoons minced garlic

1 teaspoon crushed red pepper flakes

1 (15-ounce) can chickpeas, drained (liquid reserved)

3½ teaspoons salt, divided

¼ cup dry white wine

1 pound linguine, fettuccine, or flat egg noodles

¼ cup grated Parmesan cheese

¾ cup chopped fresh Italian flat-leaf parsley

1 Heat 3 tablespoons oil in a large saucepan over medium heat. Add onion powder, rosemary, garlic, and crushed red pepper flakes. Cook, stirring, for 2 minutes. Stir in chickpeas and cook for 5 minutes.

2 Add ½ teaspoon salt, wine, and reserved chickpea liquid. Reduce heat to medium-low and simmer for 10 minutes.

3 Meanwhile, bring a large pot of water to a boil over high heat. Add pasta and remaining 3 teaspoons salt. Cook pasta according to package directions. Drain and transfer to a large serving bowl. Add chickpea mixture and toss to combine.

4 Drizzle the remaining 1 tablespoon oil over the pasta mixture. Sprinkle with Parmesan and parsley. Serve immediately.

Lasagna Florentine

The term Florentine *is used in classic French and Italian cuisine to refer to a dish containing spinach. Spinach is a healthy green; it's packed with antioxidant carotenoids, fiber, and vitamin C.*

5 cups marinara sauce, divided

1 pound whole-wheat lasagna noodles, cooked and drained, divided

3 large eggs

2 cups ricotta cheese

2 cups shredded mozzarella cheese, divided

2 cups chopped cooked spinach

½ cup chopped fresh parsley

1 teaspoon salt

¾ teaspoon ground black pepper

½ cup grated Parmesan cheese

SERVES 8	
Per Serving	
Calories	293
Fat	15g
Sodium	760mg
Carbohydrates	23g
Fiber	3g
Sugar	0g
Protein	16g

1 Preheat oven to 350°F. Oil a large baking dish or spray with non-stick cooking spray.

2 Spread 1 cup sauce on the bottom of the prepared baking dish. Cover sauce with a layer of cooked noodles.

3 In a medium bowl, combine eggs, ricotta, and 1 cup mozzarella cheese. Stir in spinach, parsley, salt, and pepper.

4 Spread half of the ricotta mixture over noodles in the dish, then top with a layer of noodles. Ladle 2 cups sauce over noodles and top with another layer of noodles.

5 Spread remaining ricotta mixture over noodles. Top with another layer of noodles, then the remaining sauce.

6 Scatter remaining 1 cup mozzarella cheese over sauce, then sprinkle Parmesan cheese over it. Bake for 1 hour 15 minutes.

7 Let lasagna cool for 10 minutes before serving.

Creamy Avocado Fettuccine

SERVES 6

Per Serving

Calories	222
Fat	10g
Sodium	679mg
Carbohydrates	25g
Fiber	5g
Sugar	2g
Protein	8g

Avocado is full of healthy fats that can help reduce the symptoms of arthritis. Healthy fats also help to produce the skin's natural oils, which keep the skin plump and hydrated.

2 tablespoons extra-virgin olive oil, divided

1 medium shallot, peeled and thinly sliced

½ medium red bell pepper, seeded and thinly sliced

½ medium green bell pepper, seeded and thinly sliced

1 cup corn kernels

1 cup black beans

¼ teaspoon ground coriander

3¾ teaspoons salt, divided

8 ounces fettuccine or linguine

2 large ripe avocados, peeled and pitted

3 cloves garlic, peeled

½ cup grated Parmesan cheese

½ cup heavy cream or half-and-half

½ teaspoon ground black pepper

¼ cup chopped cilantro

1 Heat 1 tablespoon oil in a large skillet over medium heat. Add shallot, bell peppers, corn, beans, coriander, and ¼ teaspoon salt. Sauté for 7–8 minutes until vegetables begin to soften.

2 Meanwhile, fill a large pot with water and bring to a boil over high heat. Add pasta and 3 teaspoons salt. Cook pasta for 12 minutes. Reserve ½ cup pasta cooking water before draining. Transfer pasta to a large bowl and keep warm.

3 In a food processor, combine remaining 1 tablespoon oil, avocados, garlic, Parmesan, cream, black pepper, and remaining ½ teaspoon salt. Purée until smooth.

4 Add vegetable mixture and avocado sauce to the pasta and toss to coat. Add a splash of pasta cooking water to thin and create a saucy consistency if necessary. Top with cilantro and serve warm.

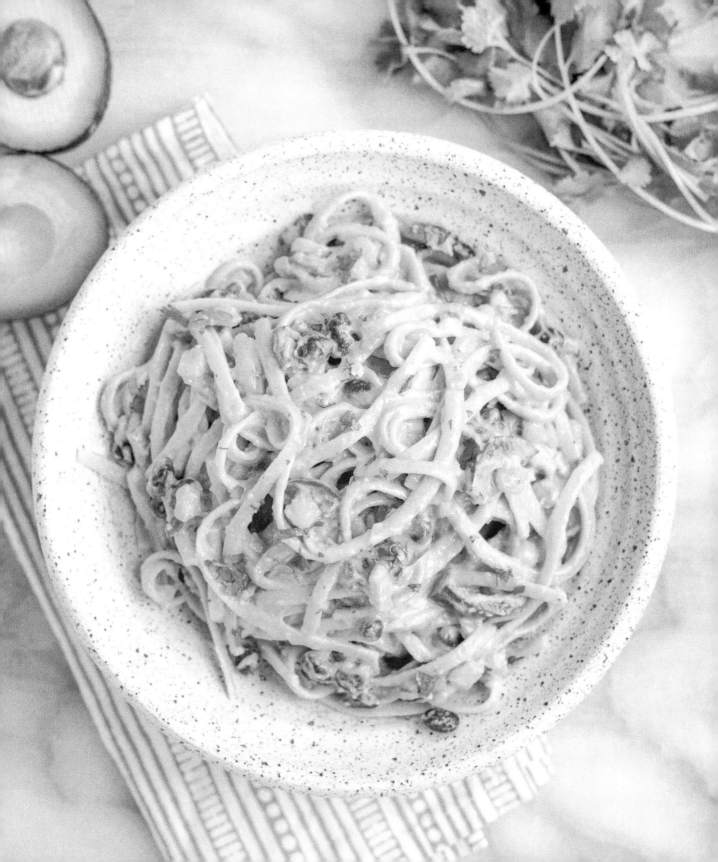

Pesto alla Trapanese

A Sicilian twist on the classic pesto, this golden version is made from blanched almonds, Parmesan, basil, and tomatoes. Almonds are a good source of plant-based protein.

16 ounces farfalle (bow-tie pasta)

3½ teaspoons salt, divided

1 cup packed fresh basil leaves

½ cup blanched almonds

½ cup grated Parmesan cheese

1 clove garlic, peeled

¾ cup canned diced tomatoes

¼ teaspoon ground black pepper

¾ cup extra-virgin olive oil

1 Bring a large pot of water to a boil over high heat. Add pasta and 3 teaspoons salt. Cook for 11 minutes, then drain. Transfer to a large bowl and keep warm.

2 Meanwhile, combine basil, almonds, Parmesan, garlic, tomatoes, pepper, and remaining ½ teaspoon salt in the bowl of a food processor. Pulse a few times, then run on low while drizzling in oil until pesto is smooth.

3 Add pesto to pasta and toss to combine. Serve warm.

Spinach and Mushroom Orzo Risotto

Earthy mushrooms and vibrant green spinach go well together in this easy shortcut risotto.

4 cups vegetable broth

1 tablespoon plant-based butter

1 tablespoon extra-virgin olive oil

1 small yellow onion, peeled and diced

2 cloves garlic, peeled and minced

16 ounces cremini mushrooms, minced

1 cup orzo

¼ teaspoon ground black pepper

⅓ cup dry white wine

5 ounces baby spinach, finely chopped

⅓ cup shredded vegan Parmesan-style cheese

1. Place broth in a medium saucepan over medium heat. Bring to a simmer, then reduce heat to low.

2. Heat plant-based butter and oil in a large saucepan over medium heat. Add onion, garlic, and mushrooms. Cook, stirring occasionally, until onion is softened, 5–7 minutes.

3. Add orzo and pepper to the large saucepan. Stir and cook for 2 minutes, then add wine. Cook until the liquid evaporates, about 1 minute.

4. Add ½ cup broth to the large saucepan and cook, stirring, until the liquid is absorbed. Repeat with the remaining broth, ½ cup at a time, waiting until the previous batch is absorbed before adding the next.

5. Remove from heat and stir in spinach and vegan cheese. Serve immediately.

SERVES 4

Per Serving

Calories	300
Fat	11g
Sodium	410mg
Carbohydrates	31g
Fiber	6g
Sugar	12g
Protein	19g

Mushroom and Herb Couscous

SERVES 6

Per Serving

Calories	200
Fat	6g
Sodium	431mg
Carbohydrates	25g
Fiber	6g
Sugar	6g
Protein	12g

Couscous is a grain made of rolled semolina (durum wheat). It's fluffy and tender, and it makes a great side dish. A ¼-cup serving of whole-wheat couscous has 3 grams of fiber.

1 cup vegetable broth

1 cup whole-wheat couscous

2 tablespoons extra-virgin olive oil

16 ounces cremini mushrooms, thinly sliced

1 small shallot, peeled and minced

3 cloves garlic, peeled and minced

¼ cup chopped fresh Italian parsley

1 tablespoon chopped fresh rosemary

1 tablespoon chopped fresh thyme

1 teaspoon salt

1. Add vegetable broth to a small saucepan and bring to a boil over high heat. Stir in couscous and remove from heat. Cover and set aside for 5 minutes, then fluff with a fork.

2. Meanwhile, heat oil in a large skillet over medium heat. Add mushrooms, shallot, and garlic. Cook, stirring occasionally, until mushrooms are tender, 6–7 minutes.

3. Add cooked couscous to the skillet and stir to combine. Remove from heat and stir in parsley, rosemary, thyme, and salt. Serve immediately.

Udon Noodle Slaw

Broccoli slaw can be found in the prepacked salad area of your grocery store's produce section. It usually contains shredded broccoli stems, carrots, and cabbage. Broccoli and cabbage are high in anti-inflammatory plant compounds.

1 (1-pound) package fresh udon noodles

1 (12-ounce) package broccoli slaw

3 tablespoons chopped pickled ginger

⅓ cup low-sodium soy sauce

2 tablespoons brown rice vinegar

1 tablespoon toasted sesame oil

1 tablespoon low-fat mayonnaise

1 tablespoon sugar

1 Bring a large pot of water to a boil over high heat. Add noodles and cook for 1 minute. Drain and rinse in cold water. Transfer to a large bowl and set aside for 10 minutes.

2 Add broccoli slaw and ginger to noodles and toss together.

3 In a small bowl, whisk together soy sauce, vinegar, sesame oil, mayonnaise, and sugar. Pour over noodle mixture and toss to coat. Serve at room temperature or refrigerate for at least 1 hour.

SERVES 4

Per Serving

Calories	216
Fat	6g
Sodium	769mg
Carbohydrates	37g
Fiber	2g
Sugar	4g
Protein	3g

UDON NOODLES

When cooking udon noodles, be sure to rinse them in cold water once they are done boiling. This helps remove the starch that clings to the strands and causes them to stick together.

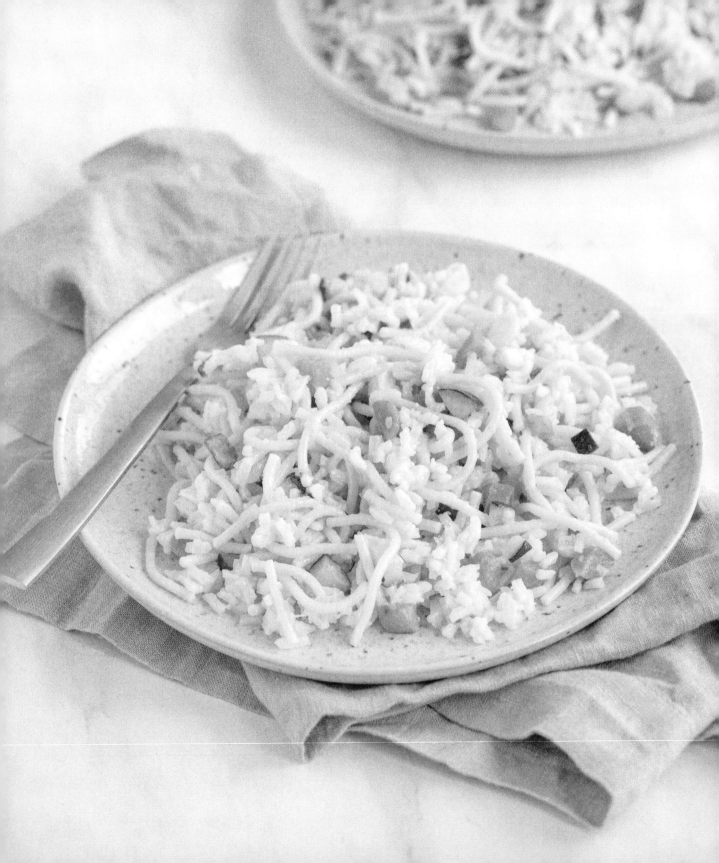

Pasta-Rice Pilaf with Vegetables

Carrots and zucchini are packed with vitamins A and C. You can switch up the vegetables with whatever you have on hand—yellow onion, squash, or celery would be good additions.

2 tablespoons extra-virgin olive oil or plant-based butter

3 medium leeks (white and light green parts only), thinly sliced

2 cloves garlic, peeled and minced

1 small zucchini, trimmed and diced

1 medium carrot, peeled and diced

5 ounces spaghetti, broken into 1" pieces

4 cups vegetable broth

1 cup long-grain rice

1. Heat oil in a large pot over medium heat. Add leeks and garlic and cook, stirring occasionally, until leeks soften, 4–5 minutes.
2. Add zucchini, carrot, and pasta. Cook, stirring constantly, until pasta browns, 1–2 minutes.
3. Stir in broth and rice. Increase heat to high and bring to a boil. Reduce heat to low, cover, and simmer for about 15 minutes until broth is absorbed. Serve warm.

SERVES 6

Per Serving

Calories	153
Fat	5g
Sodium	160mg
Carbohydrates	24g
Fiber	2g
Sugar	3g
Protein	3g

Coconut Turmeric Rice and Greens

SERVES 4

Per Serving

Calories	141
Fat	9g
Sodium	763mg
Carbohydrates	13g
Fiber	1g
Sugar	1g
Protein	2g

Turmeric is a powerful antioxidant and anti-inflammatory. The curcumin in turmeric can help prevent Alzheimer's disease and cancer as well as improve heart health. It brings a warm, earthy flavor to this satisfying side dish.

2 tablespoons extra-virgin olive oil, divided

1 small shallot, peeled and minced

3 cloves garlic, peeled and minced

1 cup long-grain rice

1 (13.5-ounce) can coconut milk

⅔ cup vegetable broth

1 teaspoon salt

1 teaspoon ground turmeric

1 bunch Swiss chard, trimmed and chopped

1. Heat 1 tablespoon oil in a large saucepan over medium heat. Add shallot and garlic. Cook, stirring occasionally, until shallot softens, 3–4 minutes.
2. Add rice, coconut milk, broth, salt, and turmeric. Increase heat to high and bring to a boil. Reduce heat to low, cover, and simmer for 15–18 minutes until the rice is tender.
3. Heat remaining 1 tablespoon oil in a medium skillet over medium heat. Sauté chard until softened, 6–7 minutes. Add to rice and stir to combine. Serve immediately.

Wild Rice Stir-Fry with Snow Peas and Broccolini

With its delicate nutty flavor and sturdy texture, wild rice makes a delicious base for any number of add-in ingredients.

½ cup water

1 tablespoon cornstarch

3 tablespoons vegetable oil

4 cloves garlic, peeled and minced

1 tablespoon minced fresh ginger

3 cups cooked wild rice

¼ pound snow peas, trimmed

1 bunch Broccolini, trimmed, cooked until crisp-tender and chopped

1 (8-ounce) can water chestnuts, drained

1 bunch scallions, trimmed and sliced

5 tablespoons hoisin sauce

3 tablespoons soy sauce

½ cup whole cashews

1 In a small bowl, whisk together water and cornstarch. Set aside.

2 Heat oil in a large wok over medium-high heat. Add garlic, ginger, and wild rice and stir-fry for 1 minute. Add snow peas, Broccolini, and water chestnuts and stir-fry for 3 minutes more. Add scallions, hoisin sauce, soy sauce, and water-cornstarch mixture. Reduce heat to medium-low and cook, covered, for 2 minutes.

3 Uncover wok and stir-fry the mixture for 2 minutes more or until vegetables are tender. Spoon onto serving plates, garnish with cashews, and serve.

SERVES 6

Per Serving

Calories	257
Fat	12g
Sodium	658mg
Carbohydrates	31g
Fiber	3g
Sugar	8g
Protein	6g

WILD RICE IS NOT A RICE?

Despite its name, wild rice is not a rice but rather is a grass native to the Great Lakes region. Typically, the rice requires thorough rinsing and lengthy cooking to tenderize the grains. But some markets now sell precooked wild rice in vacuum-sealed foil packets that requires only a few moments of reheating to ready it for the table.

Quinoa Parsley Tabbouleh

SERVES 6

Per Serving

Calories	206
Fat	11g
Sodium	303mg
Carbohydrates	22g
Fiber	2g
Sugar	4g
Protein	4g

HIGH-PROTEIN MEAL

Quinoa makes this traditional Middle Eastern dish high in protein. Add some vegetables and a bean dish to round out the protein profile of this meal. Tabbouleh is also light enough to serve as a side dish with fish, chicken, or beef.

Tabbouleh is a fresh herb salad originating from the Middle East. It usually contains bulgur, parsley, lemon juice, and olive oil. This version replaces the bulgur with protein-packed quinoa.

1 cup quinoa, rinsed and drained

2 cups low-sodium vegetable stock

¾ teaspoon salt, divided

2 small plum tomatoes

1 clove garlic, peeled and minced

¼ cup extra-virgin olive oil

3 tablespoons lemon juice

1 cup minced fresh parsley

3 scallions, trimmed and minced

1 In a medium heavy saucepan over high heat, combine quinoa, stock, and ½ teaspoon salt; bring to a boil. Reduce heat to medium-low and simmer until all liquid is absorbed, 15–20 minutes. Transfer quinoa to a large bowl and set aside to cool.

2 Halve tomatoes lengthwise and scoop out seeds into a measuring cup or small bowl. Strain and discard tomato seeds and pour tomato juice into a small bowl. Chop tomatoes into small pieces and add to quinoa.

3 Add garlic, oil, lemon juice, and remaining ¼ teaspoon salt to tomato juice. Whisk to combine.

4 Add parsley and scallions to quinoa mixture; toss well. Pour lemon mixture over quinoa mixture and mix well. Serve immediately.

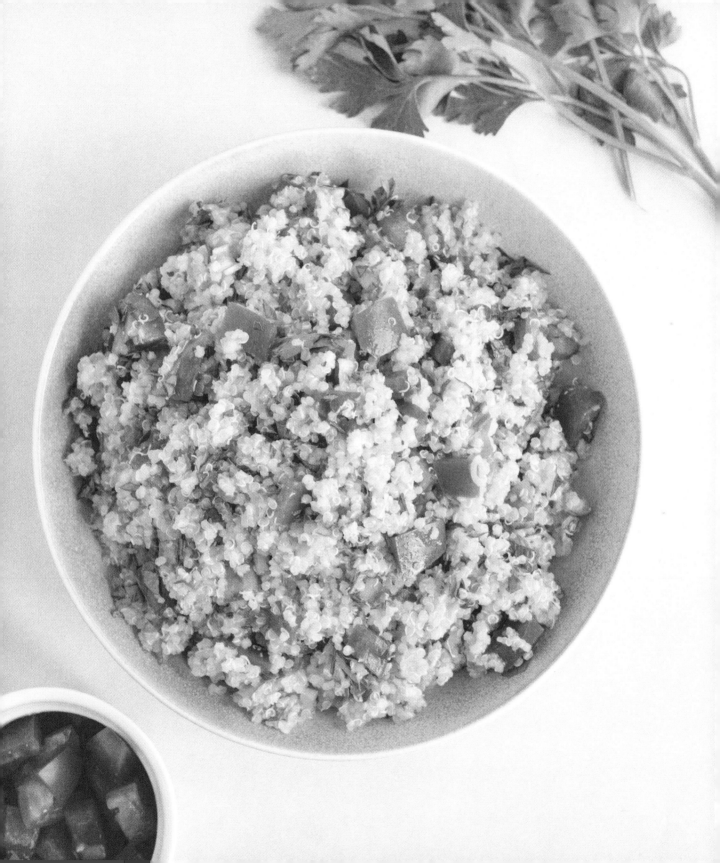

Polenta

SERVES 6

Per Serving

Calories	85
Fat	1g
Sodium	281mg
Carbohydrates	14g
Fiber	9g
Sugar	2g
Protein	5g

Polenta is a dish made from boiled whole-grain yellow or white cornmeal. It can be boiled, fried, baked, grilled, and served morning, noon, or night.

1 cup nonfat milk

2 cups low-sodium chicken stock

½ cup cornmeal

¼ cup grated Parmesan cheese

½ teaspoon ground black pepper

1 In a large heavy-bottomed saucepan, bring milk and stock to a boil over medium heat. Slowly whisk in cornmeal a bit at a time, stirring frequently, until mixture is the consistency of mashed potatoes, about 15 minutes.

2 Remove from heat, add cheese and pepper, and serve hot.

Quinoa with Sautéed Garlic

The garlic and onion in this dish provide a good amount of antioxidants—along with savory aromatic flavor. Serve this alongside grilled chicken or steak with a green salad.

1 cup quinoa, rinsed and drained

2 cups low-sodium vegetable stock

½ medium yellow onion, peeled and diced

½ teaspoon salt

¼ cup extra-virgin olive oil

6 cloves garlic, peeled and sliced

1 In a medium heavy saucepan over high heat, combine quinoa, stock, onion, and salt; bring to a boil. Reduce heat to medium-low and simmer until all liquid is absorbed, 15–20 minutes. Transfer quinoa to a large bowl and set aside to cool.

2 Heat oil in a small skillet over medium heat; sauté garlic until just crisp, but not yet brown, 1–2 minutes. Remove from heat.

3 Pour garlic and oil over quinoa; toss gently. Serve hot.

SERVES 6

Per Serving

Calories	202
Fat	11g
Sodium	206mg
Carbohydrates	22g
Fiber	2g
Sugar	2g
Protein	4g

A GLUTEN SUBSTITUTE

For gluten-intolerant individuals, quinoa is a good substitute for gluten-based grains such as couscous, a refined wheat product that also cooks quickly and is found in many Middle Eastern recipes. Quinoa is available in grain, flour, bread, and pasta form in many natural-food stores.

Shallot Walnut Herb Bread

SERVES 8

Per Serving

Calories	342
Fat	14g
Sodium	292mg
Carbohydrates	47g
Fiber	5g
Sugar	6g
Protein	7g

ANTI-INFLAMMATORY WALNUTS

Walnuts are a delicious and crunchy source of the inflammation-busting omega-3 fatty acids, and contain more omega-3s than any other nut. Walnuts can help reduce heart disease risk factors, such as high cholesterol and blood pressure.

This flavorful loaf is perfect with a cheese plate or fruit, and is an excellent source of fiber from the whole-wheat flour, shallot, and walnuts.

1 (0.25-ounce) packet yeast

3 tablespoons maple syrup, divided

1⅓ cups warm water, divided

4 tablespoons vegetable oil, divided

1 teaspoon salt

¼ teaspoon baking powder

1¾ cups all-purpose flour

1¾ cups whole-wheat flour

1 small shallot, peeled and minced

½ cup chopped walnuts

1 tablespoon minced fresh sage

1 tablespoon minced fresh thyme

1 Combine yeast, 1 teaspoon maple syrup, and ⅓ cup warm water in a small bowl. Let sit for 5 minutes.

2 To the bowl of a stand mixer, add remaining 1 cup warm water and 2⅔ tablespoons maple syrup, 3 tablespoons oil, salt, and baking powder and mix until combined. Mix in all-purpose flour and then the yeast mixture. Add whole-wheat flour, shallot, walnuts, sage, and thyme. Knead with a dough hook on low for 10 minutes.

3 Brush remaining 1 tablespoon oil on the inside of a large bowl. Place dough in bowl and turn to coat with oil. Cover and let rise in a warm place for 1–2 hours until doubled in bulk.

4 Oil a 9" × 5" loaf pan.

5 Punch down dough, then shape into a cylinder and place in the prepared pan. Cover and let rise in a warm place for 90 minutes or until doubled in size.

6 Preheat oven to 350°F.

7 Uncover bread and bake for 40 minutes. Cool in pan for 10 minutes, then transfer to a wire rack to cool completely.

CHAPTER 8

Pizza, Tacos, Wraps, and Sandwiches

Pita Pizzas with Roasted Garlic White Sauce

SERVES 4

Per Serving

Calories	478
Fat	29g
Sodium	817mg
Carbohydrates	39g
Fiber	1g
Sugar	4g
Protein	15g

ROASTED GARLIC

Once garlic is roasted, it transforms into a creamy, savory paste. Try mixing it into softened butter, spreading it on toast, or tossing it into your favorite pasta sauce.

Garlic is a potent anti-inflammatory and antifungal food. Roasting it removes the pungency of raw garlic and creates a creamy, smooth, and flavorful paste that's delicious added to sauces. Top pizzas with your favorite vegetables, like sliced olives and baby spinach or chopped tomato and onion.

1 head garlic

3 tablespoons extra-virgin olive oil, divided

2 tablespoons all-purpose flour

1 cup vegetable broth

¼ teaspoon salt

4 ounces cream cheese

2 cups shredded mozzarella cheese

4 (6") whole-wheat pita rounds

1 Preheat oven to 425°F.

2 Peel the outer papery layers from garlic and use a sharp knife to cut ¼" off the top to expose the cloves inside. Drizzle with 1 tablespoon oil and place in the center of a square of foil. Wrap foil around garlic and place directly on an oven rack. Roast for 20–30 minutes until cloves are soft. Remove from oven, loosen foil, and set aside to cool slightly.

3 Heat remaining 2 tablespoons oil in a small saucepan over medium heat. Whisk in flour and cook for 1 minute, stirring constantly, then add broth and salt. Cook, stirring, until mixture starts to thicken, 3–4 minutes.

4 Stir in cream cheese and mozzarella and cook until melted and combined, about 2 minutes.

5 Unwrap garlic and separate cloves. Squeeze the softened garlic from each clove into the saucepan. Stir to combine, then remove from heat.

6 Place pita rounds on a large ungreased baking sheet and top each with an equal amount of sauce.

7 Bake for 4–5 minutes until the pita rounds are crisp. Serve immediately.

BBQ Jackfruit Tacos

Jackfruit is a large tree fruit grown in southeast Asia, Africa, and South America. Under a thick, bumpy skin is a stringy flesh that is hearty and neutral-tasting, especially when it's slightly underripe. Jackfruit shreds easily to form a texture like pulled pork or beef and it soaks up the flavors of seasonings and sauces. It's a good source of vitamin C, potassium, and fiber, all of which can benefit heart health.

2 tablespoons extra-virgin olive oil, divided

1 small yellow onion, peeled and thinly sliced

1 medium yellow bell pepper, seeded and thinly sliced

½ teaspoon salt

1 (20-ounce) can young jackfruit, drained and shredded with a fork

1 cup barbecue sauce

½ small head red cabbage, cored and shredded

½ cup cilantro leaves

1 tablespoon lime juice

12 (6") corn tortillas

1 Heat 1 tablespoon oil in a large skillet over medium heat. Add onion, bell pepper, and salt. Cook, stirring occasionally, until soft, 5–7 minutes. Add jackfruit and cook for another 5 minutes. Stir in barbecue sauce and reduce heat to low. Cover and simmer for 15 minutes.

2 In a large bowl, combine cabbage, cilantro, lime juice, and remaining 1 tablespoon oil.

3 Place tortillas on a flat work surface. Divide jackfruit mixture among tortillas and top with cabbage mixture. Serve immediately.

SERVES 6	
Per Serving	
Calories	267
Fat	6g
Sodium	562mg
Carbohydrates	47g
Fiber	13g
Sugar	13g
Protein	6g

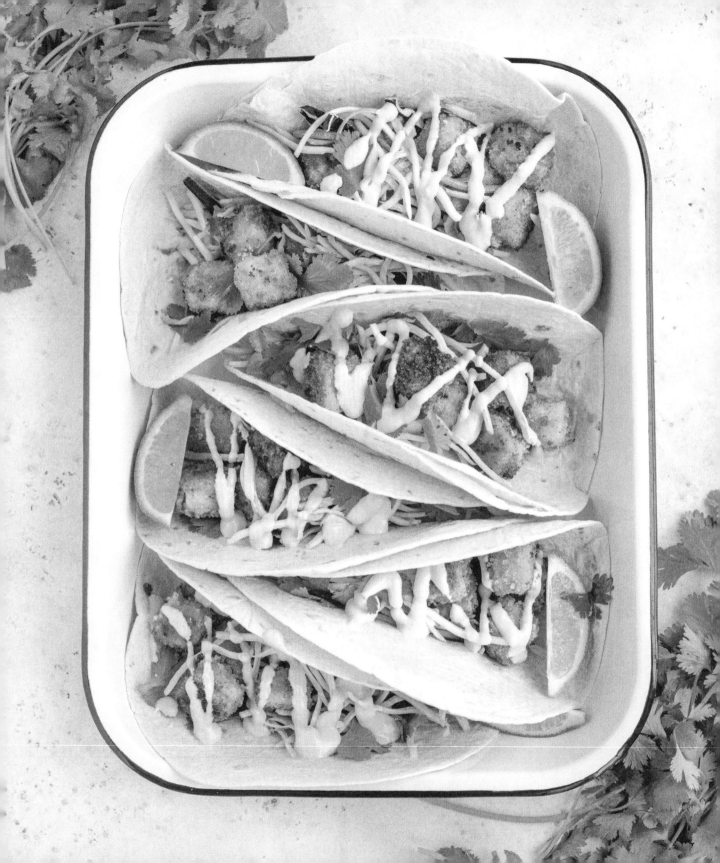

Crispy Tofu Tacos with Avocado Crema

Here's a delicious option for your taco night! Tofu is a good source of plant-based protein, and it gets nice and crispy when you press it and bake it in the oven.

1 cup almond or soy milk

½ cup all-purpose flour

1 cup panko bread crumbs

1 teaspoon garlic powder

½ teaspoon paprika

½ teaspoon salt

1 (14-ounce) package extra-firm tofu, drained, pressed, and cut into 1" cubes

8 (6") flour tortillas

1 cup broccoli slaw

1 recipe Vegan Avocado Crema (see recipe in Chapter 6)

¼ cup chopped fresh cilantro

1 Preheat oven to 400°F. Line a large baking sheet with foil or a silicone liner.

2 Place milk and flour in two separate shallow bowls. In a third shallow bowl, combine panko, garlic powder, paprika, and salt.

3 Dip each tofu cube into flour, then milk, then the panko mixture, pressing to adhere the bread crumbs.

4 Place cubes in a single layer on the prepared baking sheet. Bake for 15 minutes, then flip tofu cubes and bake for another 15 minutes or until tofu cubes are golden brown.

5 Place tortillas on a flat work surface. Divide tofu and broccoli slaw among tortillas and top with Vegan Avocado Crema and cilantro. Serve immediately.

SERVES 4

Per Serving

Calories	504
Fat	13g
Sodium	384mg
Carbohydrates	75g
Fiber	3g
Sugar	1g
Protein	19g

TOFU PRESS

To get the most liquid out of a block of tofu, invest in a tofu press. These devices effortlessly squeeze out the moisture into a tray underneath. Using a press is so much easier than wrapping tofu in towels and stacking all your heavy pans on top—and you won't miss the mess!

Cheezy Vegan Beef Burritos

SERVES 4

Per Serving

Calories	366
Fat	17g
Sodium	518mg
Carbohydrates	35g
Fiber	1g
Sugar	8g
Protein	18g

Green bell peppers are an excellent source of vitamin C, which aids in wound healing in the body.

16 ounces vegan crumbles (ground meat substitute)

1 medium green bell pepper, seeded and diced

1 (1-ounce) packet taco seasoning

½ cup water

4 (10") flour tortillas

1 cup shredded vegan Cheddar cheese substitute

1 tablespoon extra-virgin olive oil

1 Heat a large nonstick skillet over medium heat. Sauté vegan crumbles and bell pepper until crumbles have browned and the pepper is soft, 6–7 minutes. Stir in taco seasoning and water. Cook, stirring often, until sauce thickens, 3–4 minutes.

2 Place tortillas on a flat work surface. Top each with vegan crumble mixture and sprinkle with cheese substitute. Roll each tortilla tightly into a cylinder shape.

3 Wipe the skillet clean with a paper towel and place over medium-high heat. Heat oil and add burritos to the skillet. Cook 3–4 minutes until golden brown and crisp, then flip and cook for another 3 minutes. Serve warm.

Spicy Roasted Chickpea Wraps with Lemon Tahini Dressing

Roasting chickpeas gives them a hearty and crispy texture. Pair the delicious morsels with a creamy dressing and crunchy vegetables for a fun and healthy wrap.

2 tablespoons olive oil, divided

4 tablespoons lemon juice, divided

1 teaspoon honey

2 teaspoons low-sodium soy sauce, divided

2 teaspoons smoked paprika

1½ teaspoons ground cumin

1 teaspoon garlic powder

¼ teaspoon ground cayenne pepper

2 (15-ounce) cans low-sodium chickpeas, drained and rinsed

¼ cup tahini

3 tablespoons water

1 tablespoon seasoned rice vinegar

2 teaspoons minced garlic

8 (8") whole-wheat tortillas

4 cups chopped spinach or romaine lettuce

1 medium English cucumber, julienned

1 cup shredded carrots

1 Preheat oven to 400°F.

2 In a large bowl, whisk together 1 tablespoon oil, 2 tablespoons lemon juice, honey, 1 teaspoon soy sauce, paprika, cumin, garlic powder, and cayenne. Add chickpeas and stir gently to coat. Spread chickpeas onto a large ungreased baking sheet and bake for 20–25 minutes until lightly browned and crisp, stirring every 5 minutes.

3 In a small bowl, whisk together tahini, water, vinegar, minced garlic, and remaining 1 teaspoon soy sauce, 1 tablespoon oil, and 2 tablespoons lemon juice.

4 Place tortillas on a flat work surface. Top with spinach, cucumber, carrots, and chickpeas. Drizzle with tahini mixture. Roll each into a cylinder shape and serve immediately.

SERVES 4

Per Serving

Calories	652
Fat	24g
Sodium	501mg
Carbohydrates	84g
Fiber	26g
Sugar	4g
Protein	25g

RICE VINEGAR

Made from fermented rice in East Asia, rice vinegar is sweet and light, while regular vinegar is pungent and sour. It's used to sweeten sushi rice and dressings.

A Superhero Wrap-Up

SERVES 1

Per Serving

Calories	428
Fat	19g
Sodium	398mg
Carbohydrates	42g
Fiber	5g
Sugar	2g
Protein	22g

Fresh dill is full of flavonoids, which may help reduce the risk of heart attack and stroke.

1 tablespoon olive oil

1 tablespoon minced garlic

3 ounces soy "chicken" strips

¼ large red onion, peeled and thinly sliced

3 tablespoons low-fat plain Greek yogurt

2 tablespoons chopped fresh dill

½ cup julienned cucumber

½ cup julienned red bell pepper

1 (10") whole-wheat tortilla, warmed

1 Heat oil in a large skillet over medium heat. Sauté garlic, "chicken" strips, and onion for 3–4 minutes until onion wilts slightly. Transfer to a medium bowl.

2 Add yogurt, dill, cucumber, and pepper to "chicken" mixture and stir to combine.

3 Place tortilla on a flat work surface and top with mixture. Roll tortilla into a cylinder and serve.

Two-Bean Chili Wraps

Made from fermented soybeans, tempeh is an excellent source of magnesium and B vitamins and is rich in fiber, prebiotics, and protein. The isoflavones in soy are powerful antioxidants and can help to reduce cholesterol levels.

2 tablespoons olive oil

1 medium yellow onion, peeled and chopped

6 cloves garlic, peeled and chopped

2 teaspoons ground cumin

1 teaspoon ground turmeric

1 teaspoon ground cayenne pepper

16 ounces tempeh, minced

1 medium zucchini, trimmed and chopped

1 medium red bell pepper, seeded and chopped

1 (14.5-ounce) can diced tomatoes

1 (15-ounce) can kidney beans, drained and rinsed

1 (15-ounce) can cannellini beans, drained and rinsed

½ cup diced Kalamata olives

¼ teaspoon stevia

½ teaspoon salt

6 (8") whole-grain tortillas, warmed

2 cups cooked brown rice

1 medium avocado, peeled, pitted, and diced

½ cup grated Romano cheese

½ cup chopped fresh parsley

1 Heat oil in a large saucepan or Dutch oven over medium-high heat. Sauté onion until softened, 3–4 minutes. Add garlic and sauté for 30 seconds.

2 Add cumin, turmeric, and cayenne. Sauté 1 minute. Add tempeh and cook 3 minutes.

3 Stir in zucchini, bell pepper, tomatoes, beans, olives, stevia, and salt. Cover, reduce heat to medium-low, and simmer 20 minutes.

4 Place tortillas on a flat work surface and spoon rice along center of each. Top with chili, avocado, cheese, and parsley. Roll into cylinders and serve.

SERVES 6

Per Serving

Calories	662
Fat	30g
Sodium	762mg
Carbohydrates	63g
Fiber	18g
Sugar	7g
Protein	34g

A SAFE SWEETENER

Stevia helps regulate blood-sugar levels and is safe for diabetics and those needing a safe alternative sweetener. Add a little at a time, tasting as you go to determine the right level of sweetness.

Vegan BLTs with Tempeh Bacon

SERVES 4

Per Serving

Calories	359
Fat	13g
Sodium	831mg
Carbohydrates	40g
Fiber	6g
Sugar	8g
Protein	24g

Tempeh has a hearty, chewy texture and a nutty flavor. Marinating it in liquid smoke and soy sauce gives it a flavor very similar to bacon.

2 tablespoons liquid smoke

2 tablespoons soy sauce

1 tablespoon barbecue sauce

½ teaspoon garlic powder

12 ounces tempeh, thinly sliced into strips

8 (1-ounce) slices whole-wheat bread

2 tablespoons vegan mayonnaise

1 head butter lettuce

2 large ripe tomatoes, sliced

1 Whisk together liquid smoke, soy sauce, barbecue sauce, and garlic powder in a medium bowl. Add tempeh and stir to combine. Set aside to marinate for 30 minutes.

2 Heat a large nonstick skillet over medium heat. Add tempeh and cook, turning occasionally, until crisp and browned, 8–10 minutes.

3 Place 4 slices of bread on a flat surface. Spread each slice with ½ tablespoon vegan mayonnaise. Divide tempeh bacon among bread slices. Top with lettuce, tomato slices, and the remaining bread slices. Serve immediately.

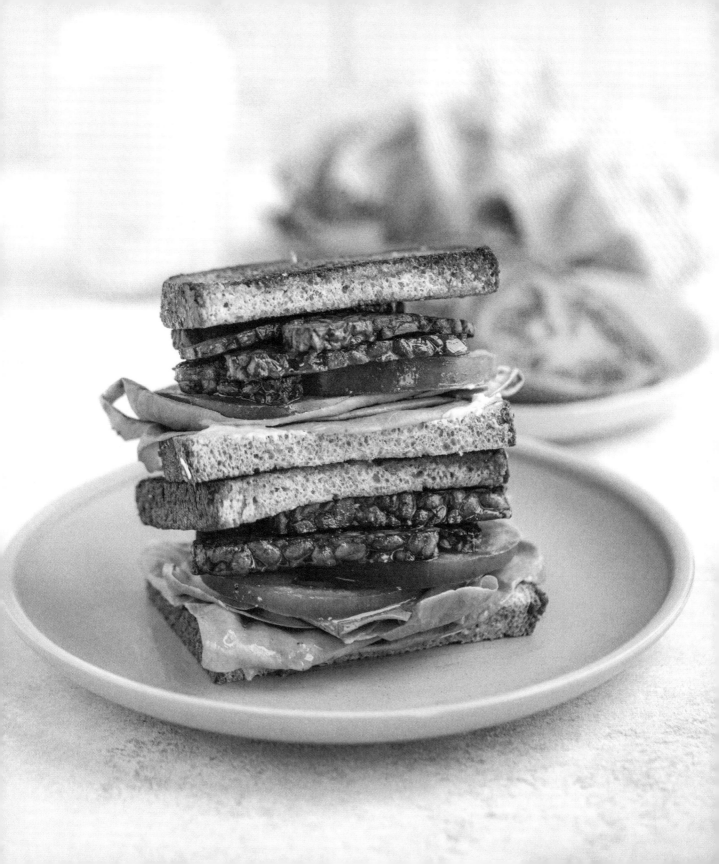

Grilled Vegetable Heros

SERVES 6

Per Serving

Calories	291
Fat	12g
Sodium	559mg
Carbohydrates	38g
Fiber	8g
Sugar	4g
Protein	8g

Eggplant is high in polyphenols, which may help diabetics process sugar more easily in the body.

1 medium eggplant, trimmed and cut into 1" slices

1 large red bell pepper, seeded and quartered

1 large Vidalia onion, peeled and quartered

2 tablespoons extra-virgin olive oil, divided

6 (8") whole-wheat tortillas

3 ounces goat cheese, crumbled

½ teaspoon ground black pepper

1 Preheat a charcoal or gas grill.

2 In a large bowl, gently toss eggplant, bell pepper, and onion with 1 tablespoon oil. Place vegetables directly on grill grate or in a grilling basket. Grill, turning often, for 10–15 minutes until tender. Transfer vegetables to a cutting board and roughly chop them.

3 Place tortillas on a flat work surface and brush with remaining 1 tablespoon oil. Divide vegetables among tortillas and top with cheese. Sprinkle with black pepper.

4 Roll each tortilla into a cylinder, cut in half, and serve immediately.

Creamy Dill Chickpea Salad Sandwiches

If you're a fan of egg or chicken salad sandwiches, you'll enjoy these chickpea salad sandwiches. The flavors of dill and mayonnaise are delicious paired with crunchy lettuce and ripe tomato slices.

3 (15-ounce) cans chickpeas, drained and rinsed

1 small shallot, peeled and minced

½ cup mayonnaise (vegan or regular)

2 tablespoons chopped fresh dill

1 tablespoon Dijon mustard

1 tablespoon white wine vinegar

½ teaspoon paprika

½ teaspoon salt

¼ teaspoon ground black pepper

12 (1-ounce) slices whole-grain bread

1 head green leaf lettuce, separated into leaves

2 medium tomatoes, thinly sliced

1 In a medium bowl, mash chickpeas into a paste using a fork. Fold in shallot, mayonnaise, dill, mustard, vinegar, paprika, salt, and pepper.

2 Place 6 slices bread on a flat work surface. Divide chickpea mixture among slices. Top with lettuce and tomatoes. Cover with remaining bread slices and serve.

SERVES 6

Per Serving

Calories	465
Fat	19g
Sodium	554mg
Carbohydrates	56g
Fiber	11g
Sugar	7g
Protein	17g

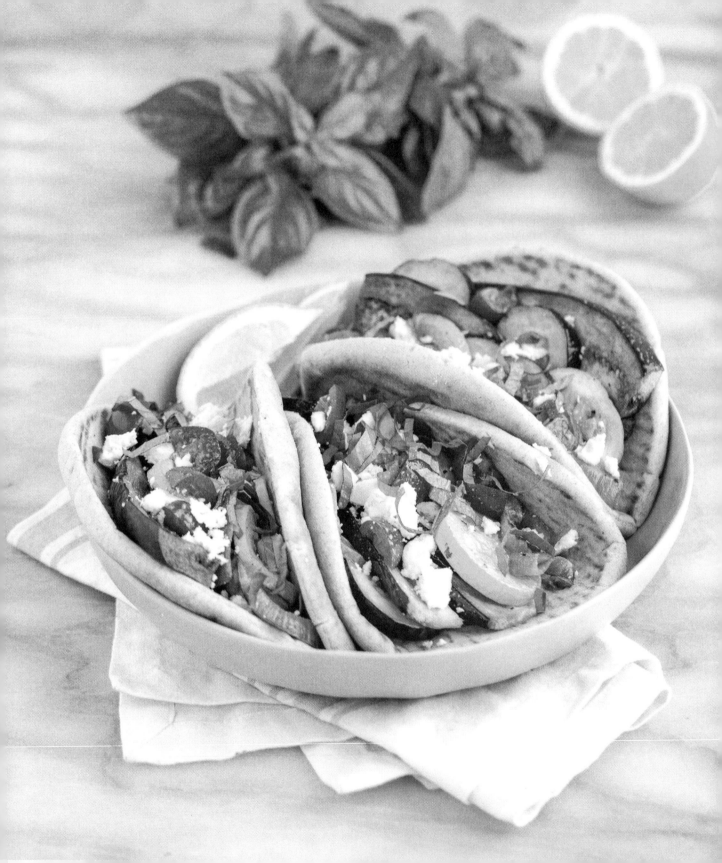

Vegetable Pitas with Feta Cheese

Roasting vegetables brings out their natural sweetness, making it an easier and tastier way to get more of them in your diet.

1 medium eggplant, trimmed and sliced lengthwise into ½" pieces

1 large zucchini, trimmed and sliced

1 large yellow squash, trimmed and sliced

1 large red onion, peeled and cut into ⅓" rings

2 tablespoons olive oil

½ teaspoon ground black pepper

6 (6") pita bread rounds

1 pint cherry tomatoes, halved

1 cup julienned fresh basil

3 ounces crumbled feta cheese

SERVES 6

Per Serving

Calories	259
Fat	8g
Sodium	380mg
Carbohydrates	37g
Fiber	6g
Sugar	8g
Protein	9g

1 Preheat oven to 375°F.

2 Brush eggplant, zucchini, yellow squash, and onion with oil and place on a rack set on a large baking sheet. Sprinkle with pepper. Roast 10 minutes, then remove from oven and flip vegetables. Roast 5–10 minutes more until tender.

3 Top pita rounds with roasted vegetables, tomatoes, basil, and cheese. Fold each pita round in half and serve immediately.

Falafel Sandwiches

Falafel is a traditional Middle Eastern dish made with chickpeas, which are high in gut-friendly fiber and a good source of plant-based iron.

SERVES 6

Per Serving

Calories	212
Fat	10g
Sodium	589mg
Carbohydrates	23g
Fiber	5g
Sugar	3g
Protein	7g

PLAIN YOGURT

When a recipe calls for sour cream, try swapping in plain yogurt instead. It's lower in fat and higher in protein, and it has a similar tart taste.

1 cup dried chickpeas

½ cup chopped red onion

3 cloves garlic, peeled

1 teaspoon salt

1 teaspoon ground black pepper

1 teaspoon ground cumin

⅛ teaspoon ground cayenne pepper

1 teaspoon baking powder

3 tablespoons all-purpose flour

3 tablespoons whole-wheat flour

2 cups vegetable oil

3 (10") pita bread rounds

6 tablespoons hummus

1 cup chopped fresh tomatoes

1 cup shredded lettuce

½ cup chopped cucumbers

6 tablespoons low-fat plain yogurt

2 tablespoons chopped fresh parsley

1. Place chickpeas in a large bowl and cover with water. Soak overnight.
2. Drain chickpeas and transfer to a food processor. Add onion, garlic, salt, black pepper, cumin, and cayenne pepper. Pulse until smooth.
3. Sprinkle baking powder and flours over the mixture and pulse again until well combined. Transfer to a covered container and refrigerate for 3 hours.
4. Heat oil in a deep fryer or large pot to 375°F.
5. Shape chickpea mixture into small balls and fry 4–5 at a time until browned and crispy, 2–3 minutes. Drain on paper towels.
6. Cut pita rounds in half and open them to create a pocket in each half. Spread the inside of a pita pocket with hummus, stuff 3–4 falafel balls into it, and top with tomatoes, lettuce, and cucumbers. Drizzle yogurt over the top and sprinkle with parsley. Repeat with remaining ingredients.
7. Serve immediately.

Balsamic Portobello Burgers

Portobello mushrooms are of the same variety as cremini mushrooms; they're allowed to mature and grow larger. They have a dense, meaty texture and taste great grilled.

4 large portobello mushroom caps, stems and gills removed

2 tablespoons extra-virgin olive oil, divided

½ cup balsamic vinegar

1 large yellow onion, peeled and thinly sliced

½ teaspoon salt

4 (1.75-ounce) brioche buns

4 (1-ounce) slices provolone cheese

1 Place a grill pan over medium heat.
2 Brush mushroom caps with 1 tablespoon oil. Grill, turning halfway, until mushrooms are tender, 4–5 minutes.
3 Place balsamic vinegar in a small saucepan over medium heat. Bring to a boil, then reduce heat to low and simmer for 10 minutes or until reduced by half.
4 Heat remaining 1 tablespoon oil in a medium skillet over medium heat. Add onion and salt. Cook, stirring occasionally, until onion browns and caramelizes, 15–20 minutes.
5 Place the bottom of a bun on a plate. Top with a mushroom cap, a spoonful of caramelized onions, a drizzle of reduced balsamic vinegar, and a slice of cheese. Repeat with the remaining ingredients. Serve immediately.

SERVES 4

Per Serving

Calories	465
Fat	22g
Sodium	723mg
Carbohydrates	48g
Fiber	3g
Sugar	10g
Protein	16g

BALSAMIC GLAZE

To save time, you can buy premade balsamic glaze at most grocery stores. Look for it near the vinegar shelves. Once opened, a bottle of balsamic glaze lasts a long time in the refrigerator.

Mushroom Burgers with Roasted Garlic Aioli

Adding mushrooms to burgers is a great way to add vegetables to a meal while also adding flavor! Using a grill pan means you can enjoy these flavorful burgers anytime. But you can also cook them on an outdoor grill.

CHOOSING MAYONNAISE

When shopping for mayonnaise at the grocery store, look for one made with olive oil. This ensures you'll get a higher amount of heart-healthy fats than you would from regular mayonnaise.

1 head garlic

1 tablespoon extra-virgin olive oil

2 pounds 93% lean ground beef

16 ounces cremini mushrooms, minced

1 teaspoon Worcestershire sauce

½ teaspoon salt

¼ teaspoon ground black pepper

½ cup mayonnaise

6 (2-ounce) hamburger buns

1 Preheat oven to 425°F.

2 Peel the outer papery layers from garlic and use a sharp knife to cut ¼" off the top to expose the cloves inside. Drizzle with oil and place in the center of a square of foil. Wrap foil around garlic and place directly on an oven rack. Roast for 20–30 minutes until cloves are soft. Remove from oven, loosen foil, and set aside to cool slightly.

3 In a medium bowl, combine ground beef, mushrooms, Worcestershire sauce, salt, and pepper. Form into six equal-sized patties.

4 Heat a grill pan over medium heat. Place patties on the pan and cook for 5 minutes per side.

5 Unwrap garlic and separate cloves. Squeeze the softened garlic from each clove into a small bowl. Add mayonnaise and mash together with a fork until combined.

6 Serve burgers on buns, topped with aioli.

CHAPTER 9

Plant-Based Proteins

Spicy Thai Basil Tofu

SERVES 4

Per Serving

Calories	290
Fat	13g
Sodium	801mg
Carbohydrates	30g
Fiber	2g
Sugar	1g
Protein	14g

RICE OPTIONS

There are two main varieties of long-grain rice—basmati and jasmine. Basmati has a dry and fluffy texture, while jasmine rice is soft and sticky. Choose whichever texture you'd like best to go with the dish you're serving.

Thai basil is slightly different from the garden-variety basil you'll often see in most grocery stores or home gardens. It has a purple stem and a spicier flavor than regular basil, making it a great addition to dishes like this one.

1 cup vegetable broth

¼ cup soy sauce

1 tablespoon fish sauce

1 tablespoon light brown sugar

1 (14-ounce) package extra-firm tofu, drained and pressed, cut into 1″ cubes

2 tablespoons cornstarch

2 tablespoons extra-virgin olive oil

3 cloves garlic, peeled and minced

2 small shallots, peeled and minced

2 medium jalapeño peppers, seeded and chopped

2 cups cooked long-grain rice

1 cup julienned Thai basil leaves

1   In a medium bowl, whisk together broth, soy sauce, fish sauce, and brown sugar. Set aside.

2   Place tofu in a large bowl and sprinkle with cornstarch. Toss to coat.

3   Heat oil in a large nonstick skillet over medium-high heat. Add tofu cubes, garlic, shallots, and jalapeños. Cook, stirring occasionally, until tofu is crisp and shallots and jalapeños soften, 8–10 minutes.

4   Pour broth mixture into the skillet and reduce heat to medium-low. Cook, stirring occasionally, for 10–12 minutes until sauce thickens and glazes tofu.

5   Serve with rice and garnish with basil.

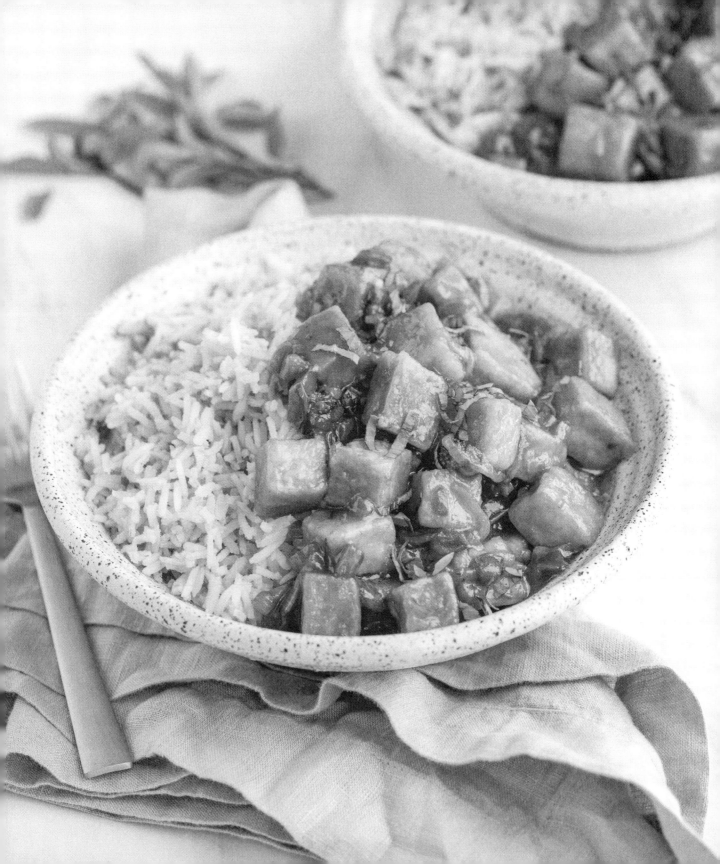

Crispy Sweet Chili Tofu Sticks with Broccoli Slaw

SERVES 4

Per Serving

Calories	327
Fat	14g
Sodium	561mg
Carbohydrates	36g
Fiber	2g
Sugar	12g
Protein	14g

ALL ABOUT PANKO

Panko is a Japanese-style bread crumb made from crustless white bread. It is much lighter and crunchier than regular bread crumbs, making it perfect for breading and frying.

Sweet chili sauce is made with red chili peppers, rice wine vinegar, garlic, and a sweetener (usually sugar or honey). It's typically used as a dipping sauce for spring rolls, but it can also be used as a delicious sauce for chicken or tofu.

1 cup panko bread crumbs

½ teaspoon garlic powder

½ teaspoon salt

¼ cup cornstarch

1 (14-ounce) package extra-firm tofu, drained, pressed, and sliced into ½" planks

2 tablespoons extra-virgin olive oil

½ cup sweet chili sauce

1 (12-ounce) package broccoli slaw

1 Place panko, garlic powder, and salt in a shallow bowl and stir to combine. Place cornstarch in another shallow bowl. Dip tofu pieces into cornstarch, shake off excess, then dip into the panko mixture, pressing to adhere.

2 Heat oil in a large nonstick skillet over medium heat. Add tofu and cook for 6–8 minutes per side until golden brown and crispy on both sides. Transfer to a large bowl.

3 Add chili sauce and toss to coat. Serve with broccoli slaw.

Sesame Tofu

Five-spice powder is a mix of five spices that are a big part of Chinese cuisine. It typically includes Sichuan pepper, cinnamon, fennel, star anise, and cloves.

½ cup rice flour

⅛ teaspoon five-spice powder

1 teaspoon sesame oil

1 large egg or ¼ cup egg substitute

¾ cup sesame seeds

1 (14-ounce) package extra-firm tofu, drained and cubed

½ cup peanut oil

½ cup teriyaki sauce

4 cups cooked white rice

¼ cup sliced scallions

1 In a shallow bowl, mix flour and five-spice powder. In another shallow bowl, whisk together sesame oil and egg. Place sesame seeds in a third shallow bowl.

2 Dredge tofu in flour mixture, then dip in egg mixture and toss in sesame seeds to coat. Lay tofu on a platter in a single layer and let dry for 10 minutes.

3 Heat oil in a large skillet over medium-high heat and pan-fry tofu until crispy, 8–10 minutes.

4 Drain tofu on paper towels and transfer to a large bowl. Add teriyaki sauce and toss gently to coat. Serve over rice and garnish with scallions.

SERVES 4

Per Serving

Calories	671
Fat	30g
Sodium	379mg
Carbohydrates	78g
Fiber	5g
Sugar	12g
Protein	21g

Spicy Peanut Tofu Stir-Fry

SERVES 4

Per Serving

Calories	399
Fat	21g
Sodium	396mg
Carbohydrates	38g
Fiber	4g
Sugar	5g
Protein	14g

Zucchini slices are an easy, delicious, and healthy choice to add to stir-fry dishes. They cook quickly, have a sweet taste, and are rich in the antioxidants lutein and zeaxanthin.

1 cup vegetable broth

¼ cup creamy peanut butter

1 teaspoon chili-garlic sauce

1 tablespoon soy sauce

2 cloves garlic, peeled and minced

2 teaspoons seasoned rice vinegar

2 tablespoons sesame oil, divided

1 (14-ounce) package extra-firm tofu, drained, pressed, and cut into 1" cubes

2 tablespoons cornstarch

2 medium zucchini, trimmed and sliced into thin half-moons

1 cup shredded carrots

2 cups cooked long-grain rice

½ cup sliced scallions

1 Combine broth, peanut butter, chili-garlic sauce, soy sauce, garlic, vinegar, and 1 tablespoon sesame oil in a small saucepan over medium heat. Cook, whisking occasionally, until sauce thickens, 4–5 minutes. Remove from heat and set aside.

2 Place tofu in a large bowl and sprinkle with cornstarch. Toss to coat.

3 Heat remaining 1 tablespoon oil in a large nonstick skillet over medium heat. Add tofu cubes, zucchini, and carrots. Cook, stirring occasionally, until tofu is crisp and zucchini and carrots soften, 8–10 minutes.

4 Pour peanut sauce into the skillet and toss to combine. Serve over rice and garnish with scallions.

Ma Po Tofu

Ma Po is a popular Chinese dish of tofu in a spicy red sauce with ground meat. In this version, soy crumbles replace the meat for a delicious plant-based meal.

3 tablespoons vegetable oil

4 cloves garlic, peeled and minced

1 (1") piece fresh ginger, peeled and thinly sliced

3 tablespoons black bean–garlic sauce

2 tablespoons soy sauce

1 tablespoon garlic-chili paste

1 cup low-sodium vegetable stock

1 tablespoon cornstarch

1 tablespoon sugar

1 (14-ounce) package firm tofu, drained, pressed, and cubed

6 ounces vegan crumbles (ground meat substitute)

2 bunches scallions, trimmed and cut diagonally

1 Heat oil in a large wok or skillet over medium heat. Add garlic and ginger and stir-fry for 30 seconds. Stir in black bean–garlic sauce, soy sauce, and garlic-chili paste. Cook, stirring constantly, for 1 minute.

2 In a small bowl, stir together stock, cornstarch, and sugar. Add to wok. Stir in tofu and vegan crumbles and stir-fry until sauce thickens and tofu is heated through, 5–7 minutes. Add scallions, stir-fry for 2 minutes more, and serve.

SERVES 4

Per Serving

Calories	270
Fat	18g
Sodium	651mg
Carbohydrates	15g
Fiber	2g
Sugar	8g
Protein	12g

VARIETIES OF TOFU

Tofu is available in a variety of types, defined by firmness. The most common types are silken, soft, medium, firm, extra-firm, and super-firm. Silken tofu is best used in sauces, dressings, and desserts, providing a thick and creamy texture. Firmer varieties hold their shape in cooking, and they are good for stir-frying, pan-frying, and baking. Extra-firm and super-firm tofu make the best crispy cubes.

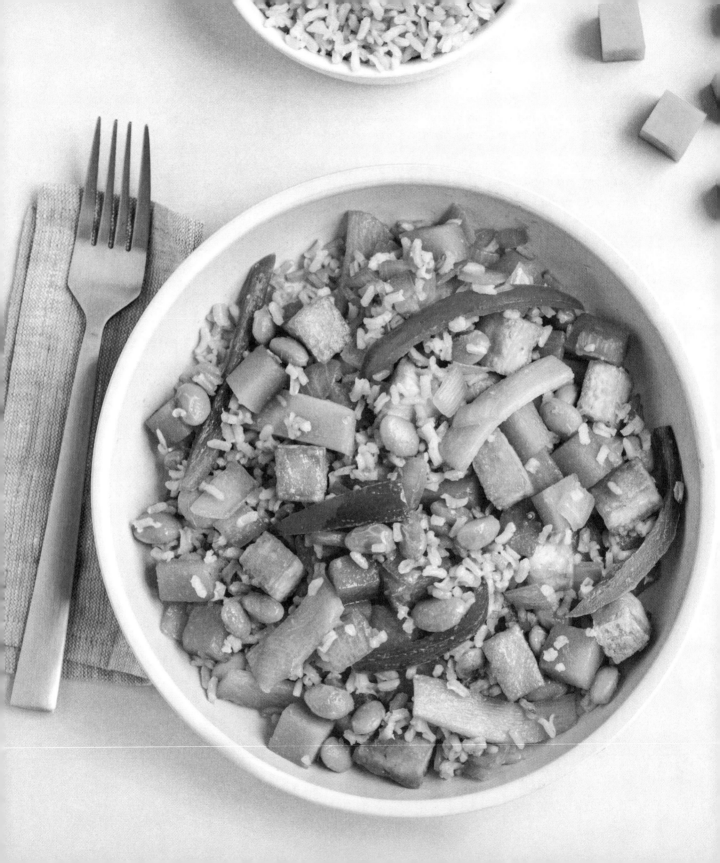

Asian Stir-Fried Rice

Edamame are immature soybeans in the pod, which are served steamed or boiled. The pods are discarded, and the beans can be eaten alone or mixed into dishes. They're a great source of plant-based iron.

3 tablespoons canola oil

8 ounces firm tofu, drained and cubed

3 cloves garlic, peeled and minced

1 medium yellow onion, peeled and diced

1 tablespoon minced fresh ginger

1 cup cubed butternut squash

1 cup shelled edamame

1 (8-ounce) can sliced bamboo shoots, drained

2 long green chilies, thinly sliced

2 cups cold cooked short-grain brown rice

3 tablespoons soy sauce

1 Heat oil in a large wok or skillet over medium-high heat. Add tofu and stir-fry for 5–7 minutes until it starts to brown. Remove tofu from the wok and set aside.

2 Add garlic, onion, and ginger and stir-fry for 1 minute. Add squash and edamame and stir-fry for 2 minutes.

3 Stir in tofu, bamboo shoots, chilies, rice, and soy sauce. Cover the wok and cook the mixture for about 5 minutes until squash is tender. During cooking, check that the mixture does not get too dry; add up to ½ cup water as needed, stirring it in well. Serve hot.

SERVES 4

Per Serving

Calories	348
Fat	16g
Sodium	802mg
Carbohydrates	36g
Fiber	4g
Sugar	4g
Protein	15g

WHY CHILL THE RICE?

If you don't chill cooked rice before stir-frying, the grains will clump together and become mushy; they're also likely to absorb too much oil while cooking. Besides, stir-frying is a great way to use up leftover rice in your refrigerator. This recipe calls for short-grain brown rice, which is somewhat sticky but provides a delicious texture and flavor to the dish. Any leftover rice, though, will work.

Butter Tofu

SERVES 4

Per Serving

Calories	319
Fat	17g
Sodium	612mg
Carbohydrates	29g
Fiber	3g
Sugar	2g
Protein	12g

In traditional Indian-style butter chicken, cream creates a silky-smooth sauce. In this vegan version, coconut milk replaces the cream.

1 (14-ounce) block extra-firm tofu, drained and pressed

3 tablespoons olive oil, divided

1 tablespoon cornstarch

1 teaspoon salt, divided

1 medium yellow onion, peeled and thinly sliced

1 tablespoon grated fresh ginger

2 cloves garlic, peeled and minced

2 teaspoons garam masala

½ teaspoon curry powder

½ teaspoon ground coriander

2 tablespoons tomato paste

1 (13.5-ounce) can coconut milk

2 cups cooked long-grain rice

½ cup chopped fresh cilantro

1 Preheat oven to 400° F. Line a large baking sheet with parchment paper or a silicone baking mat.

2 Rip tofu into 2" chunks and place in a large bowl. Add 1 tablespoon oil, cornstarch, and ½ teaspoon salt. Toss to coat, then spread onto the prepared baking sheet. Bake for 30–35 minutes, turning halfway through, until tofu is golden and crispy.

3 Heat remaining 2 tablespoons oil in a large saucepan over medium heat. Sauté onion until softened, 3–4 minutes. Add ginger and garlic and sauté for 1 minute. Add garam masala, curry powder, coriander, remaining ½ teaspoon salt, tomato paste, and coconut milk. Bring to a simmer, then reduce heat to low. Simmer for 10 minutes. Stir in tofu.

4 Serve over rice and garnish with cilantro.

Tofu Mac and Cheese

This grown-up version of a comfort-food favorite includes a surprise ingredient: Spanish olives, also called manzanilla olives. *These firm, pale green morsels have a briny taste that adds a delicious salty flavor.*

3 heads fresh spinach, stemmed and roughly chopped

2 tablespoons olive oil

2½ tablespoons all-purpose flour

2 cups nonfat milk

3 cups cooked pasta shells

3 ounces goat cheese, crumbled

3 ounces firm tofu, drained and cubed

¼ cup chopped Spanish olives

1 small shallot, peeled and minced

3 cloves garlic, peeled and minced

½ teaspoon ground black pepper

1   Preheat oven to 350°F. Spray a large baking dish with nonstick cooking spray.

2   Heat 1" water in a large saucepan over medium-high heat. Place a steamer insert in the pan and add spinach. Cover and steam for 3 minutes. Transfer spinach to a medium bowl and set aside.

3   Heat oil in a medium saucepan over medium heat, then add flour. Stir mixture constantly to form a roux. Whisk in milk and cook until thickened, about 3 minutes, to make a white sauce. Pour half of the sauce into prepared baking dish.

4   Layer pasta, spinach, cheese, tofu, olives, shallot, garlic, and pepper over sauce, then top with remaining sauce.

5   Cover and bake for 15–20 minutes until heated through. Uncover and bake for 5–10 minutes longer until lightly browned. Serve.

SERVES 6

Per Serving

Calories	277
Fat	13g
Sodium	315mg
Carbohydrates	27g
Fiber	1g
Sugar	4g
Protein	13g

GOAT CHEESE

Goat cheese, or chèvre, is made from goat's milk. It is lower in lactose, is easier to digest, and contains more vitamins and minerals than cheese made from cow's milk.

Creamy Chipotle Tempeh with Cilantro Lime Rice

IS RINSING RICE NECESSARY?

Rinsing rice before cooking removes any excess starch clinging to the grains. The result? The grains stay more separate when cooked, making your rice less mushy.

Canned chipotle peppers have a great smoky flavor and impart a delicious spiciness to the vegan sauce.

2 cups vegetable broth

1 cup basmati rice

¼ cup chopped fresh cilantro leaves

4 teaspoons lime juice, divided

1 teaspoon grated lime zest, divided

2 tablespoons olive oil, divided

¾ cup vegan mayonnaise

1 chipotle pepper from a can of chipotles in adobo sauce

2 cloves garlic, peeled

1 teaspoon maple syrup

¼ teaspoon salt

12 ounces tempeh, thinly sliced

2 medium red bell peppers, seeded and sliced

1 Add broth to a medium saucepan. Bring to a boil over high heat, then add rice. Reduce heat to low, cover, and simmer for 15 minutes or until liquid is absorbed. Fluff with a fork and stir in cilantro, 2 teaspoons lime juice, and ½ teaspoon lime zest.

2 In a blender, combine 1 tablespoon oil, vegan mayonnaise, chipotle pepper, garlic, maple syrup, salt, and remaining 2 teaspoons lime juice and ½ teaspoon lime zest. Purée until smooth and set aside.

3 Heat remaining 1 tablespoon oil in a large skillet over medium heat. Add tempeh and bell pepper and cook, turning occasionally, until tempeh is golden and crispy and pepper strips are tender, about 8 minutes.

4 To serve, divide rice mixture among four plates. Top with tempeh and bell pepper strips. Drizzle with chipotle sauce.

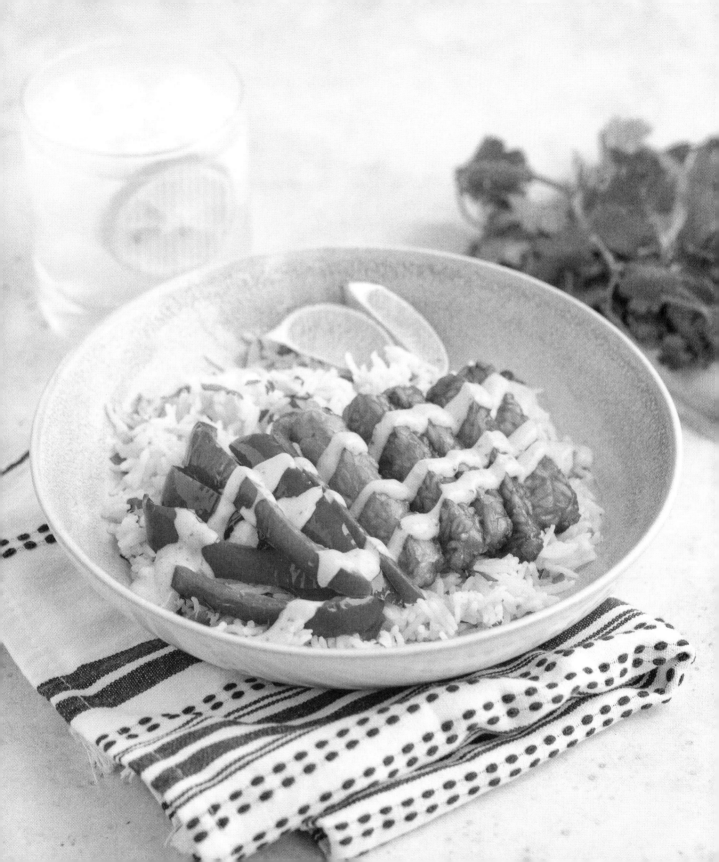

BBQ Tempeh with Couscous and Broccolini

Broccolini is a hybrid of regular broccoli and Chinese kale, with long, thin stalks. It has a sweeter, less bitter taste than broccoli.

SERVES 4

Per Serving

Calories	395
Fat	10g
Sodium	557mg
Carbohydrates	54g
Fiber	10g
Sugar	13g
Protein	22g

12 ounces tempeh, thinly sliced

1 cup barbecue sauce

1 cup vegetable broth

1 cup whole-wheat couscous

1 tablespoon extra-virgin olive oil

2 bunches Broccolini, trimmed

1 Combine tempeh and barbecue sauce in a large bowl and set aside to marinate for at least 30 minutes.
2 Place broth in a small saucepan over high heat and bring to a boil. Add couscous. Remove from heat, stir, and cover. Set aside for 5 minutes, then fluff with a fork.
3 Heat oil in a large nonstick skillet over medium-high heat. Add Broccolini and cook, stirring occasionally, until tender-crisp, 6–7 minutes. Transfer to a plate and cover with foil.
4 Return skillet to medium heat. Add tempeh and barbecue sauce. Cook, stirring occasionally, for 5 minutes.
5 To serve, divide couscous, Broccolini, and barbecue tempeh among four plates.

Curried "Meatballs" in Pita

Sweet and spicy mango chutney can be found in most grocery stores in the Indian or Southeast Asian section. Mangoes are loaded with vitamin A, which is essential for healthy eyesight.

1 tablespoon canola oil

1 cup diced tomatoes

½ cup chopped yellow onion

1 (9-ounce) package soy "meatballs"

½ cup chopped fresh cilantro

2 tablespoons mango chutney

1 tablespoon Indian curry powder

1 teaspoon ground turmeric

¼ teaspoon salt

1 cup low-fat plain yogurt

2 (10") whole-wheat pita rounds

SERVES 2	
Per Serving	
Calories	493
Fat	13g
Sodium	1,102mg
Carbohydrates	60g
Fiber	10g
Sugar	23g
Protein	34g

1 Heat oil in a large skillet over medium heat and sauté tomatoes and onion until softened, about 5 minutes.

2 Cut "meatballs" in half and add them to the skillet, stirring well and cooking until they are heated through, about 3 minutes. Stir in cilantro, chutney, curry powder, turmeric, and salt. Cook for 2 minutes more, then stir in yogurt. Cook for 3 minutes, stirring occasionally.

3 To serve, cut pita rounds in half and spoon the mixture evenly inside. Alternatively, you can wrap the "meatballs" up in the pita, tucking one end up to prevent dripping.

Sweet and Sour "Meatballs" over Brown Rice

SERVES 4

Per Serving

Calories	590
Fat	25g
Sodium	1,024mg
Carbohydrates	70g
Fiber	5g
Sugar	34g
Protein	21g

VEGETARIAN "MEATBALLS"

Although you can make a meatball-type product at home with a mixture of such ingredients as cereals, cheeses, and/ or grains, most well-stocked markets offer heat-and-serve "meat-balls" made from soy proteins. Look for them in the specialty foods section. Your friends and family may never notice the difference between these and the ground beef originals.

Vegan meatballs are typically made out of soy, pea, or rice protein (or a combination of these). For this recipe, choose precooked "meatballs" that just need to be heated through.

1 (20-ounce) can pineapple chunks in juice, drained (reserve 1 cup juice)

½ cup water

⅓ cup soy sauce

¼ cup white vinegar

3 tablespoons sugar

2 tablespoons cornstarch

2 teaspoons sesame oil

2 tablespoons canola oil

1 (9-ounce) package soy "meatballs"

1 large red bell pepper, seeded and diced

1 medium zucchini, trimmed and diced

1 bunch scallions, trimmed and sliced diagonally

2 teaspoons minced garlic

1 cup cashews

2 cups cooked brown rice

1 Combine pineapple juice, water, soy sauce, vinegar, sugar, cornstarch, and sesame oil in a medium bowl and whisk to combine. Set aside.

2 Heat canola oil in a large skillet or wok over medium heat. Add "meatballs" and stir-fry for 2 minutes. Add pineapple, pepper, zucchini, scallions, and garlic and stir-fry for 2 minutes.

3 Pour in pineapple juice mixture and stir well to coat all ingredients. Cook, stirring often, for 2 minutes more or until the sauce thickens slightly. Remove from heat and stir in the cashews. Serve over rice.

Vegan Meatloaf Cups

Meatloaf is traditionally cooked in a loaf pan and can take close to an hour to bake. This version cooks in a muffin tin and is finished baking in about 20 minutes. Swapping vegan ground meat for the beef is a great way to add plant-based protein to your weeknight meals.

1 cup ketchup

½ cup light brown sugar

1 teaspoon soy sauce

½ teaspoon dry mustard

1¼ cups plain bread crumbs

¼ cup soy milk or almond milk

½ teaspoon dried parsley

½ teaspoon onion powder

1 pound vegan crumbles (ground meat substitute)

1 Preheat oven to 400°F. Grease a twelve-cup muffin tin or line with paper liners.

2 In a small bowl, combine ketchup, brown sugar, soy sauce, and mustard. Whisk to combine.

3 In a large bowl, combine bread crumbs, milk, parsley, onion powder, vegan crumbles, and 2 tablespoons of the ketchup mixture. Use your hands to combine well.

4 Divide vegan meat mixture into twelve equal-sized balls, and place a ball in each well of the muffin tin. Smooth tops to create a flat surface.

5 Spoon 1 teaspoon of the ketchup mixture over the top of each cup. Reserve remaining sauce to be served on the side.

6 Bake for 20 minutes. Serve hot.

SERVES 6

Per Serving

Calories	350
Fat	9g
Sodium	790mg
Carbohydrates	52g
Fiber	3g
Sugar	11g
Protein	17g

SILICONE MUFFIN TIN LINERS

If you tend to bake often with muffin tins, invest in a set of reusable silicone muffin tin liners. These nonstick liners are easy to clean, and you don't even need a muffin tin to use them. They're firm enough to stand up on their own when placed on a baking sheet.

Stuffed Bell Peppers

SERVES 6

Per Serving

Calories	178
Fat	3g
Sodium	675mg
Carbohydrates	31g
Fiber	8g
Sugar	14g
Protein	7g

Stuffed peppers typically contain lean meat (such as beef or turkey), vegetables, and a fiber-rich whole grain in the stuffing. This recipe uses soy "meat" crumbles for a vegan option.

2 large green bell peppers

2 large red bell peppers

2 large yellow bell peppers

2 cups vegan crumbles (ground meat substitute)

¼ cup Grape-Nuts cereal

½ cup cooked brown rice

½ cup diced yellow onion

½ cup diced carrots

½ cup diced celery

2½ cups tomato sauce, divided

¾ teaspoon salt

½ teaspoon ground black pepper

1. Preheat oven to 350°F.
2. Cut bell peppers in half through the stems and discard seeds, stems, and membranes. Lay pepper halves in a large ungreased baking dish.
3. In a large bowl, mix together vegan crumbles, cereal, rice, onion, carrots, celery, and ½ cup tomato sauce. Season mixture with salt and black pepper.
4. Stuff each pepper half with a scoop of the vegan crumble mixture, mounding it on top.
5. Pour remaining 2 cups tomato sauce over tops of stuffed peppers. Cover dish with foil and bake for 45 minutes or until peppers are fork-tender. Serve hot.

CHAPTER 10

Beans and Lentils

Baked Beans

SERVES 6

Per Serving

Calories	338
Fat	3g
Sodium	405mg
Carbohydrates	65g
Fiber	8g
Sugar	19g
Protein	13g

Fiber- and iron-rich beans make a healthy side dish to serve at your next get-together.

4 cups cooked white beans

1 cup sliced yellow onion

4 slices turkey bacon, chopped

1 teaspoon dry mustard

½ cup light brown sugar

½ cup maple syrup

2 tablespoons ketchup

½ teaspoon salt

1 teaspoon ground black pepper

1½ cups water

1 Preheat oven to 350°F.
2 Place beans in a large shallow ungreased baking dish. Top with onion and bacon.
3 Combine mustard, brown sugar, maple syrup, ketchup, salt, pepper, and water in a medium bowl and whisk to combine. Pour mixture over beans.
4 Cover dish and bake for 2 hours. Uncover and bake for 15 minutes more. Serve warm.

Tuscan White Bean Skillet

This one-dish meal is loaded with fiber from the beans and vegetables, and full of the sun-drenched Tuscan flavors of sun-dried tomatoes, basil, and oregano.

2 tablespoons extra-virgin olive oil

4 (3-ounce) hot Italian vegan sausages, thinly sliced into rounds

1 medium yellow onion, peeled and diced

2 cloves garlic, peeled and minced

¼ cup oil-packed sun-dried tomatoes, drained and chopped

½ teaspoon salt

¼ teaspoon ground black pepper

½ teaspoon dried basil

½ teaspoon dried oregano

1 (14-ounce) can artichoke hearts, drained and chopped

1 (14.5-ounce) can petite-diced tomatoes

2 (15-ounce) cans white cannellini beans, drained and rinsed

1 head kale, stems removed and leaves chopped

1 Heat oil in a large skillet over medium heat. Add vegan sausages and cook, stirring occasionally, until golden brown on both sides, 8–10 minutes. Transfer to a plate and keep warm.

2 Return skillet to medium heat and add onion, garlic, sun-dried tomatoes, salt, pepper, basil, and oregano. Cook, stirring occasionally, for about 5 minutes until onion softens.

3 Add artichokes, diced tomatoes, beans, and kale to the skillet. Cook for 5–7 minutes, stirring occasionally, until the kale has wilted. Add vegan sausage back into the skillet and stir until combined and warmed through, about 3 minutes. Serve hot.

SERVES 4

Per Serving

Calories	582
Fat	29g
Sodium	1,182mg
Carbohydrates	52g
Fiber	15g
Sugar	8g
Protein	29g

CANNED ARTICHOKES

Artichokes are available packed in brine or oil. For most recipes, brined artichokes do best. When artichokes are packed in oil, seasonings such as basil and oregano are added, which doesn't always match the flavor of the rest of the recipe.

Refried Pinto Beans

SERVES 4

Per Serving

Calories	183
Fat	7g
Sodium	524mg
Carbohydrates	23g
Fiber	8g
Sugar	1g
Protein	7g

This homemade version of refried beans, a popular restaurant food usually served alongside tacos and enchiladas, is made with heart-healthy olive oil.

2 tablespoons olive oil

½ cup diced yellow onion

1 clove garlic, peeled and minced

1 (15-ounce) can pinto beans, undrained and mashed, divided

1 cup water, divided

1 teaspoon salt

1 Heat oil in a medium skillet over medium heat. Sauté onion until softened, 3–4 minutes. Add garlic and sauté for 30 seconds. Stir in half of the mashed beans. Cook, stirring, for 2 minutes.

2 Add ½ cup water and remaining beans and stir to combine.

3 Stir in salt and remaining ½ cup water. Cook for 10 minutes, stirring often. Serve warm or at room temperature.

Spinach and Black Bean Enchiladas

Here's an easy weeknight meal you can pull together quickly. Lots of fiber makes these enchiladas filling and satisfying.

1 (10-ounce) package frozen spinach, thawed and squeezed

6 scallions, trimmed and thinly sliced

1 (15-ounce) can black beans, drained and rinsed

15 ounces ricotta cheese

½ cup sour cream

1 teaspoon salt

1 (28-ounce) can enchilada sauce

12 (6") flour tortillas

2 cups shredded mozzarella cheese

1. Preheat oven to 375°F.
2. In a large bowl, combine spinach, scallions, beans, ricotta, sour cream, and salt.
3. Pour a small amount of enchilada sauce into the bottom of a large ungreased baking dish. Place tortillas on a flat work surface.
4. Spoon ¼ cup of the spinach mixture into the center of each tortilla. Roll to close and place seam side down in the baking dish. Pour remaining sauce over the top and sprinkle with mozzarella cheese.
5. Bake for 20–30 minutes until cheese is melted and bubbly. Serve hot.

SERVES 6

Per Serving

Calories	505
Fat	16g
Sodium	1,346mg
Carbohydrates	59g
Fiber	10g
Sugar	5g
Protein	30g

WHAT TYPE OF TORTILLA IS BEST?

Tortillas come in many different sizes and are usually made from wheat flour or corn. Flour tortillas can be made from white or whole-wheat flour, which has more fiber. Corn tortillas are more fragile and are usually best for light tacos. For heartier dishes like enchiladas, flour tortillas hold up better under sauce and cheese.

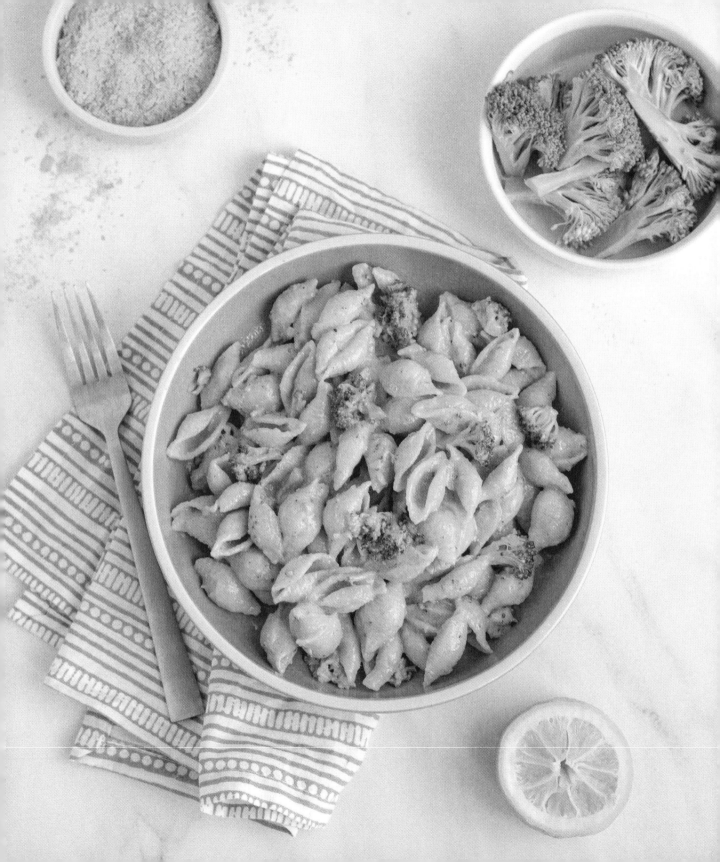

White Bean Macaroni and Cheeze

Nutritional yeast is a type of inactive yeast that is grown specifically for use as a food product or seasoning. While it's low in sodium and calories, it provides a cheesy, umami-rich flavor to vegan recipes. Nutritional yeast is high in protein and vitamin B$_{12}$ and contains powerful antioxidants that can reduce your risk of disease.

1 pound elbow macaroni or other small pasta shape

3½ teaspoons salt, divided

1 large head broccoli, cut into florets

1 (15-ounce) can white beans, drained and rinsed

½ cup vegetable broth

2 tablespoons lemon juice

2 tablespoons melted vegan butter

⅓ cup nutritional yeast

2 cloves garlic, peeled

½ teaspoon onion powder

¼ teaspoon ground black pepper

SERVES 6	
Per Serving	
Calories	299
Fat	3g
Sodium	240mg
Carbohydrates	49g
Fiber	16g
Sugar	3g
Protein	19g

1 Fill a large pot with water and bring to a boil over high heat. Add pasta and 3 teaspoons salt. Cook for 6 minutes. Add broccoli and cook for 4 minutes more. Reserve ½ cup pasta cooking water before draining. Drain pasta and broccoli, then return to the pot and set aside.

2 Place beans, broth, lemon juice, vegan butter, nutritional yeast, garlic, onion powder, pepper, and remaining ½ teaspoon salt in a blender or food processor. Purée until smooth.

3 Pour sauce over pasta and broccoli and stir to combine. Add a splash of pasta cooking water to thin the sauce if necessary. Serve immediately.

Red Beans and Rice

SERVES 4

Per Serving

Calories	290
Fat	4g
Sodium	621mg
Carbohydrates	49g
Fiber	9g
Sugar	1g
Protein	14g

This happy marriage of legume and grain is a Caribbean favorite that will feed a family without leaving anyone hungry. You can substitute brown rice for extra fiber.

1 tablespoon olive oil

¼ cup diced celery

¼ cup diced yellow onion

¼ cup diced green bell pepper

1 clove garlic, peeled and minced

¼ cup diced cooked ham

2 cups cooked red kidney beans

½ teaspoon dried thyme

¼ teaspoon cayenne pepper

¾ cup water

½ teaspoon salt

2 cups cooked white rice

1. Heat oil in a large skillet over medium-high heat. Sauté celery, onion, bell pepper, and garlic for 5–6 minutes until onion is translucent.
2. Add ham, beans, thyme, cayenne pepper, water, and salt. Reduce heat to medium-low and simmer for 45 minutes. Serve beans over rice.

Succotash

Lima beans are one of the best plant-based sources of iron, containing a quarter of the daily requirement in a single serving.

2 large ears corn, shucked

1 teaspoon olive oil

1 large yellow onion, peeled and diced

1 large red bell pepper, seeded and diced

½ teaspoon ground black pepper

12 ounces frozen baby lima beans, thawed

1 tablespoon all-purpose flour

½ cup nonfat milk

½ cup low-sodium vegetable stock

1 Place corn in a medium saucepan and cover with water. Bring to a boil over high heat. Immediately remove from heat, cover, and set aside for 5 minutes. Remove corn from water and use a sharp knife to cut kernels from cobs.

2 Heat oil in a large saucepan over medium heat. Add onion and sauté until light golden in color, about 6 minutes. Add bell pepper and sauté for 1 minute. Season with black pepper.

3 Add beans and corn, sprinkle with flour, and stir. Whisk in milk and stock and reduce heat to low. Simmer for 20–30 minutes until beans and vegetables are tender.

4 Serve warm or at room temperature.

SERVES 6

Per Serving

Calories	149
Fat	1g
Sodium	21mg
Carbohydrates	28g
Fiber	4g
Sugar	8g
Protein	7g

CORN ON THE COB

Fresh corn on the cob can be found in most grocery stores from May through October. When shopping for fresh corn, choose cobs with bright green husks that are tightly wrapped.

Ribollita

MIREPOIX

The holy trinity of French cooking, mirepoix, is a combination of finely diced onion, carrot, and celery that's used as a base in many dishes such as soups and roasts.

Popular in Tuscany, ribollita is a hearty vegetable stew thickened with bread. Traditionally, it was made using leftover soup and bread, but it's easy to make from scratch.

6 tablespoons extra-virgin olive oil, divided

1 medium yellow onion, peeled and diced

2 medium carrots, peeled and diced

2 stalks celery, trimmed and diced

3 cloves garlic, peeled and minced

1 teaspoon salt

¼ teaspoon ground black pepper

1 (15-ounce) can cannellini beans, drained and rinsed

1 (15-ounce) can chickpeas, drained and rinsed

1 (14.5-ounce) can diced tomatoes

6 cups vegetable broth

1 tablespoon fresh rosemary leaves

1 tablespoon fresh thyme leaves

1 head Tuscan kale, stems removed and chopped

½ (14-ounce) loaf Italian or French bread, torn into chunks, divided

1 Heat 4 tablespoons oil in a large Dutch oven or other oven-safe pot over medium heat. Add onion, carrots, celery, garlic, salt, and pepper. Sauté for 6–8 minutes until vegetables soften.

2 Add cannellini beans, chickpeas, tomatoes, broth, rosemary, thyme, kale, and half of the bread chunks. Increase heat to medium-high and bring to a boil. Reduce heat to medium-low and simmer for 20 minutes.

3 Preheat oven to 400°F.

4 Lay remaining bread chunks over the top of the soup and drizzle with remaining 2 tablespoons oil. Bake until bread is crisp, about 10 minutes. Serve immediately.

Edamame

Edamame makes a great snack, containing plenty of protein and fiber to help you feel full between meals. If you can find fresh edamame in your grocery store, use it instead of frozen.

6 cups water

½ teaspoon salt

1 pound frozen edamame in pods

1 Combine water and salt in a large saucepan. Bring to a boil over medium-high heat.
2 Add edamame and return to a boil. Cook for 5 minutes. Drain edamame and rinse with cold water.
3 Serve warm or cool.

SERVES 6	
Per Serving	
Calories	98
Fat	4g
Sodium	117mg
Carbohydrates	6g
Fiber	4g
Sugar	1g
Protein	10g

Dal

Yellow split peas have a nutty flavor that is milder than that of green split peas. They're a great source of magnesium, which is not only anti-inflammatory, but can also combat depression and insomnia.

1 tablespoon olive oil

6 cloves garlic, peeled and minced

¼ Scotch bonnet chili pepper, seeded and minced

1 cup dried yellow split peas

4 cups low-sodium vegetable stock

1 Heat oil in a medium saucepan over medium-high heat. Sauté garlic and chili for 1 minute.
2 Add peas and stock; bring to a boil. Reduce heat to low and simmer for 1½–2 hours until peas are tender. Serve warm.

SERVES 6	
Per Serving	
Calories	164
Fat	3g
Sodium	21mg
Carbohydrates	26g
Fiber	11g
Sugar	4g
Protein	8g

Lentil-Stuffed Peppers

SERVES 6

Per Serving

Calories	481
Fat	7g
Sodium	213mg
Carbohydrates	75g
Fiber	30g
Sugar	10g
Protein	30g

FABULOUS FETA

Feta cheese originates from Greece. It's made from sheep's or goat's milk (or a combination of the two) and aged in brine. Its crumbly texture makes it perfect for topping salads, wraps, and pasta dishes.

Unlike other types of lentils, red lentils are split in half, so they take the shortest time to cook.

1 tablespoon olive oil

2 medium yellow onions, peeled and diced

2 stalks celery, trimmed and diced

2 medium carrots, peeled and minced

3 cups dried red lentils

4 cups low-sodium vegetable stock, divided

6 large bell peppers

6 sprigs fresh oregano, stemmed and chopped

3 ounces feta cheese, crumbled

1 teaspoon ground black pepper

1 Heat oil in a large saucepan over medium heat. Add onions, celery, and carrots; sauté for 5 minutes, then add lentils and 1 cup stock. Simmer for 15–20 minutes until the lentils are fully cooked. Transfer to a large bowl and set aside.

2 Cut off the tops of bell peppers and remove seeds (reserve tops with stems). Place peppers in a large saucepan that will hold them all in one layer. Add remaining 3 cups stock. Cover and simmer over medium heat for 10 minutes, then remove from heat. Drain peppers and place them on a large platter or individual serving dishes.

3 Add oregano, cheese, and black pepper to the lentil mixture and stir to combine. Divide mixture among bell peppers, mounding the filling in each one. Top each pepper with a reserved pepper top. Serve immediately.

Curried Red Lentils and Tomatoes

Red lentils create a smooth and creamy texture when cooked and pair nicely with curry and turmeric. And their lovely orangey hue makes this a beautiful dish.

2 tablespoons extra-virgin olive oil

1 large yellow onion, peeled and diced

2 small jalapeño peppers, seeded and diced

3 cloves garlic, peeled and minced

3 tablespoons minced fresh ginger

1 teaspoon salt

1 teaspoon curry powder

1 teaspoon ground turmeric

¼ teaspoon ground cinnamon

¼ teaspoon ground cumin

1½ cups dried red lentils

3 cups vegetable broth

1 (13.5-ounce) can coconut milk

1 pint cherry tomatoes, quartered

1 cup chopped fresh cilantro leaves

SERVES 6	
Per Serving	
Calories	274
Fat	7g
Sodium	477mg
Carbohydrates	39g
Fiber	16g
Sugar	4g
Protein	14g

1 Heat oil in a large saucepan or Dutch oven over medium-high heat. Add onion, jalapeños, garlic, ginger, salt, curry powder, turmeric, cinnamon, and cumin. Cook, stirring occasionally, until onion softens, 5–7 minutes.

2 Add lentils, broth, and coconut milk to the pan. Bring to a boil, then reduce heat to low and simmer until lentils are tender, 20–25 minutes.

3 Remove from heat and stir in tomatoes and cilantro. Serve warm.

Black Lentil and Sweet Potato Bowls

HARISSA PASTE

Usually containing red chilies, harissa paste is peppery and smoky. It also has garlic, vinegar, lemon juice, and spices. This North African staple can be used as a marinade for meat or seafood or as a spicy dressing for vegetables. It's a great way to add heat and flavor to recipes.

While other varieties of lentils can get mushy once cooked, beluga lentils retain their shape and keep a nice al dente texture.

2 cups dried black beluga lentils

3 teaspoons salt, divided

2 pounds sweet potatoes, peeled and cut into 1" cubes

5 tablespoons olive oil, divided

1 tablespoon honey

3 tablespoons red wine vinegar

½ teaspoon ground coriander

2 tablespoons harissa paste

½ teaspoon ground black pepper

2 pints cherry tomatoes, halved

1 cup chopped fresh cilantro leaves

1 Bring a large pot of water to a boil over high heat. Add lentils and 2 teaspoons salt and reduce heat to medium-low. Simmer for about 30 minutes until lentils are tender. Drain and transfer lentils to a large bowl; set aside.

2 Preheat oven to 425°F.

3 Spread sweet potatoes on a large ungreased baking sheet and drizzle with 1 tablespoon oil. Toss to coat and sprinkle with remaining 1 teaspoon salt. Bake for about 30 minutes until browned and fork-tender.

4 Meanwhile, whisk together honey, vinegar, coriander, harissa, pepper, and remaining 4 tablespoons oil in a small bowl.

5 To serve, divide lentils, sweet potatoes, and cherry tomatoes among four bowls. Drizzle with dressing and top with cilantro.

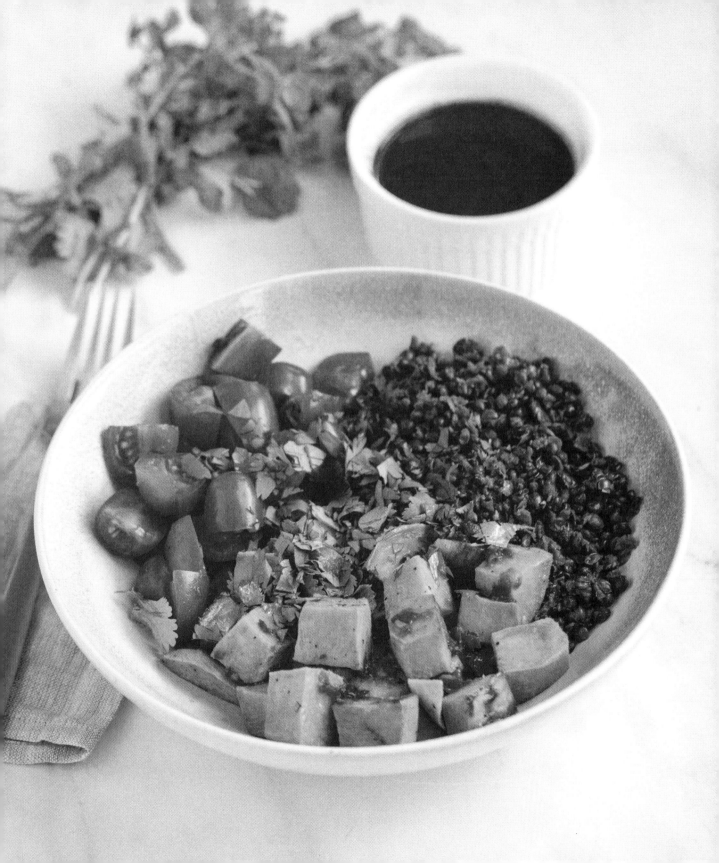

Lentil Sloppy Joes

SERVES 6

Per Serving

Calories	369
Fat	6g
Sodium	696mg
Carbohydrates	64g
Fiber	5g
Sugar	11g
Protein	14g

This recipe can also be made in an electric pressure cooker or Instant Pot®. Use the sauté function for step 1, then cover the pot and pressure cook on high for 20 minutes.

1 tablespoon extra-virgin olive oil

1 medium yellow onion, peeled and diced

2 cloves garlic, peeled and minced

1 cup dried green lentils

2 cups vegetable broth

¼ cup tomato sauce

1 tablespoon maple syrup

1 tablespoon soy sauce

½ teaspoon chili powder

½ teaspoon smoked paprika

½ teaspoon salt

12 slider hamburger buns

1 small white onion, peeled and sliced

1   Heat oil in a large saucepan or Dutch oven over medium-high heat. Sauté yellow onion until softened, 3–4 minutes. Add garlic and sauté for 30 seconds.

2   Add lentils and broth and bring to a boil. Reduce heat to low, cover, and simmer for 20–30 minutes until lentils are tender.

3   Remove from heat and stir in tomato sauce, maple syrup, soy sauce, chili powder, smoked paprika, and salt.

4   Serve on buns with slices of white onion.

CHAPTER 11

Chicken, Beef, Pork, and Seafood

Asian Sesame Chicken Skewers

SERVES 8

Per Serving

Calories	138
Fat	6g
Sodium	322mg
Carbohydrates	1g
Fiber	0g
Sugar	0g
Protein	20g

Black sesame seeds are small, flat, and oily seeds that are a good source of copper and manganese, essential for cell functioning and metabolism. White sesame seeds can be used instead if you can't find black. Or try an eye-catching combination of the two.

½ cup low-sodium chicken stock

¼ cup plus 2 tablespoons chopped fresh cilantro, divided

2 tablespoons tamari or low-sodium soy sauce

2 tablespoons sesame oil

2 cloves garlic, peeled and minced

¼ teaspoon hot pepper sauce

1½ pounds boneless, skinless chicken breasts, cut into ½" strips

2 tablespoons black sesame seeds

1 Place twenty-four wooden skewers in a baking pan filled with water to soak for at least 30 minutes.

2 In a medium bowl, combine stock, ¼ cup cilantro, tamari, sesame oil, garlic, and hot sauce and whisk until blended.

3 Add chicken strips to the marinade, stir to coat, and cover. Refrigerate for 15 minutes.

4 Preheat broiler. Lightly oil a broiler rack and position it about 4" from the heat source.

5 Remove chicken from marinade and discard marinade. Thread one strip on a presoaked wooden skewer. Thread remaining chicken on remaining skewers. (Threading the strips in the form of an S will help them stay on the skewers.)

6 Place skewers on the preheated broiler rack and broil for 3 minutes. Turn skewers over and broil for another 3–4 minutes until chicken is no longer pink.

7 Remove from oven and sprinkle with sesame seeds and remaining 2 tablespoons cilantro. Serve hot.

Zesty Pecan Chicken and Grapes

Chopped pecans add a crispy coating that keeps the chicken moist and tender. Pecans are also high in heart-healthy fats.

¼ cup chopped pecans

1 teaspoon chili powder

¼ cup olive oil

1½ pounds boneless, skinless chicken breasts

6 cups salad greens

12 ounces green grapes, halved

1 Preheat oven to 400°F. Place a wire rack on a large baking sheet.

2 In a blender, blend pecans and chili powder. While the blender is running, pour in oil until thoroughly combined. Transfer mixture to a shallow bowl.

3 Coat chicken with pecan mixture and place on the prepared racked baking sheet. Bake for 30–35 minutes until the internal temperature reaches 165°F. Remove chicken from oven and thinly slice.

4 Divide greens among six plates. Top with chicken slices and grapes. Serve immediately.

SERVES 6

Per Serving

Calories	264
Fat	13g
Sodium	101mg
Carbohydrates	8g
Fiber	2g
Sugar	5g
Protein	29g

TOASTING NUTS FOR FRESHER FLAVOR AND CRISPNESS

To wake up the natural flavor of nuts, heat them on the stovetop or in the oven for a few minutes. On the stovetop, spread the nuts in a dry skillet and toast over medium heat until their natural oils come to the surface, about 3–5 minutes. In the oven, spread the nuts in a single layer on an ungreased baking sheet and toast for 5–10 minutes at 350°F until the oils are visible. Cool nuts to room temperature before serving.

Ginger Orange Chicken Breast

SERVES 4

Per Serving

Calories	216
Fat	8g
Sodium	399mg
Carbohydrates	4g
Fiber	0g
Sugar	3g
Protein	32g

WORKING WITH CHICKEN

Boneless, skinless chicken breasts are available in many forms: fresh, frozen, marinated, seasoned, and even pre-cooked. Use fresh boneless, skinless breasts available in the meat section of your grocer. Choose a good, reputable brand and check the freshness date.

Serve this chicken warm with stir-fried vegetables and brown rice. It's also good chilled, sliced, and added to a crisp green salad.

4 (5-ounce) boneless, skinless chicken breasts

½ teaspoon salt

½ teaspoon ground black pepper

2 tablespoons butter

2 cloves garlic, peeled and minced

2 tablespoons grated fresh ginger

2 teaspoons grated orange zest

½ cup orange juice

1 Season chicken with salt and pepper.

2 Melt butter in a large nonstick skillet over medium-high heat. Cook chicken, turning once, until browned, about 8 minutes per side. Transfer chicken to a plate and keep warm.

3 Add garlic to the pan and cook for 1 minute, stirring frequently to prevent burning. Add ginger, orange zest, and juice, and bring to a simmer. Return chicken and any reserved juices to the pan and cook until the internal temperature of chicken reaches 165°F, 4–5 minutes. Serve hot.

Spicy Chicken Burgers

You can substitute ground turkey or pork for the chicken. Make the burgers as spicy as you like by adding more or less hot pepper sauce.

1 pound ground chicken

¼ cup finely chopped yellow onion

¼ cup finely chopped red bell pepper

1 teaspoon minced garlic

¼ cup thinly sliced scallions

½ teaspoon hot pepper sauce

1 teaspoon Worcestershire sauce

½ teaspoon salt

½ teaspoon ground black pepper

1 Preheat broiler.

2 Combine all ingredients in a medium bowl, mixing lightly. Form mixture into four equal-sized patties. Place patties on an ungreased broiler pan or baking sheet.

3 Broil patties for 4–5 minutes per side until firm through the center and the juices run clear. Transfer to a plate and tent with foil to keep warm. Allow to rest 2 minutes before serving.

SERVES 4

Per Serving

Calories	189
Fat	11g
Sodium	399mg
Carbohydrates	2g
Fiber	0g
Sugar	1g
Protein	21g

Chicken à la King

SERVES 4	
Per Serving	
Calories	350
Fat	5g
Sodium	332mg
Carbohydrates	49g
Fiber	2g
Sugar	4g
Protein	27g

Old-school Chicken à la King, a delicious combination of chicken, peas, and mushrooms, is a creamy, comforting meal and a great way to use up leftovers. Try it with turkey breast instead of chicken if that's what you have on hand.

1 (10.5-ounce) can low-fat condensed cream of chicken soup

¼ cup nonfat milk

½ teaspoon Worcestershire sauce

1 tablespoon low-fat mayonnaise

¼ teaspoon ground black pepper

2 cups frozen peas and pearl onions, thawed

1 cup sliced mushrooms

½ pound chopped cooked chicken breast

16 ounces egg noodles, cooked, drained, and kept warm

1 Combine soup, milk, Worcestershire sauce, mayonnaise, and pepper in a medium saucepan over medium-high heat. Bring to a boil, then reduce heat to medium-low.

2 Add peas and pearl onions, mushrooms, and chicken. Simmer for 8–10 minutes until vegetables and chicken are heated through.

3 Serve over noodles.

Chicken with Curry and Apricot Sauce

A sweet and creamy sauce is the star of this dish. The combination of sweet fruit and warm spices makes it a natural for a cool fall evening.

4 (5-ounce) boneless, skinless chicken breasts

½ teaspoon salt

½ teaspoon ground black pepper

¼ cup vegetable oil

1 cup sliced red onion

3 cloves garlic, peeled and minced

1 cup low-sodium chicken broth

2 teaspoons curry powder

1 cup apricot preserves

1 cup low-fat plain Greek yogurt

SERVES 4	
Per Serving	
Calories	545
Fat	17g
Sodium	408mg
Carbohydrates	59g
Fiber	1g
Sugar	51g
Protein	40g

1 Season chicken with salt and pepper.

2 Heat oil in a large nonstick skillet over medium-high heat. Cook chicken until lightly browned, 4–5 minutes per side. Transfer chicken to a plate and tent with foil to keep warm.

3 Reduce heat to medium-low and add onion. Cook until soft, 3–4 minutes, stirring occasionally. Add garlic and stir to combine. Add broth, curry powder, and apricot preserves; bring to a simmer and cook until thickened, about 5 minutes.

4 Return chicken and any accumulated juices to the pan and cook until the chicken is cooked through, about 5 minutes. Remove skillet from heat. Transfer chicken to a serving plate and keep warm. Add yogurt to the pan and stir to combine.

5 Ladle sauce over the chicken and serve immediately.

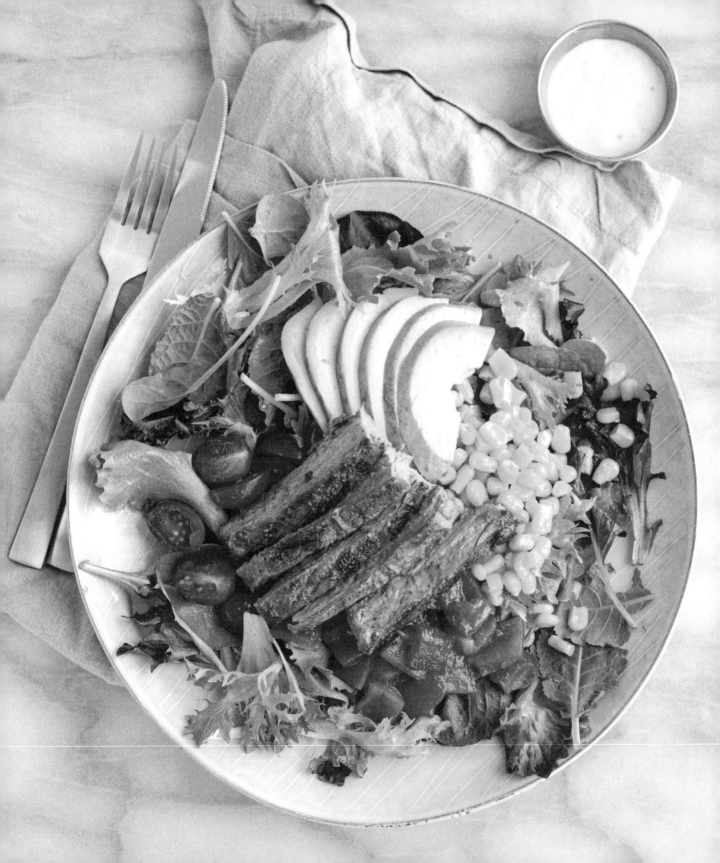

Flank Steak Salad with Roasted Corn and Peppers

Fresh corn on the cob can be easily cooked in the oven, and you don't even need to remove the husks. The corn steams from the inside out, making it tender and sweet.

4 medium ears corn, unhusked, silk trimmed

2 large red bell peppers

1 (2-pound) flank steak

2 teaspoons Montreal steak seasoning

½ teaspoon salt

½ teaspoon ground black pepper

1 (16-ounce) package spring greens mix

2 medium avocados, peeled, pitted, and sliced

1 pint cherry tomatoes, halved

½ cup ranch salad dressing

1 Preheat oven to 400°F.

2 Place corn directly on an oven rack. Roast for 30 minutes. Place bell peppers on an ungreased baking sheet and roast for 12 minutes.

3 Slice bell peppers and remove seeds. Peel corn and slice kernels off the cobs.

4 Heat a grill pan over medium heat.

5 Season steak with steak seasoning, salt, and black pepper and cook for 4 minutes per side. Transfer to a cutting board and let rest for 3 minutes. Cut diagonally across the grain into thin slices. Set aside.

6 Divide greens among six plates. Top with corn, bell peppers, steak, avocado slices, and tomatoes. Drizzle with dressing and serve immediately.

SERVES 6

Per Serving

Calories	532
Fat	30g
Sodium	636mg
Carbohydrates	28g
Fiber	7g
Sugar	5g
Protein	38g

STEAK CUTS FOR GRILLING

Lean meats are great for grilling. Fatty cuts of meat can drip grease, which causes flare-ups that can burn your food. Look for top sirloin, flank, or tenderloin steaks.

Chicken and Green Bean Stovetop Casserole

SERVES 4

Per Serving

Calories	225
Fat	5g
Sodium	269mg
Carbohydrates	23g
Fiber	2g
Sugar	4g
Protein	22g

This is a dressed-up version of a popular Thanksgiving side dish. With the addition of chicken and rice, it stands alone as a meal.

1 (10.5-ounce) can low-fat condensed cream of chicken soup

¼ cup nonfat milk

2 teaspoons Worcestershire sauce

1 teaspoon low-fat mayonnaise

½ teaspoon onion powder

¼ teaspoon garlic powder

¼ teaspoon ground black pepper

1 (4-ounce) can sliced water chestnuts, drained

2½ cups frozen green beans, thawed

1 cup sliced mushrooms

½ pound chopped cooked chicken breast

1⅓ cups cooked brown rice

1 Combine soup, milk, Worcestershire sauce, mayonnaise, onion powder, garlic powder, and pepper in a medium saucepan over medium-high heat. Bring to a boil, then reduce heat to medium-low.

2 Add water chestnuts, green beans, mushrooms, and chicken. Simmer 8–10 minutes until vegetables and chicken are heated through.

3 Serve over rice.

Soy-Glazed Steak with Mango Salsa

If you can't find fresh mango, use frozen mango. Thaw and dice the chunks into small pieces. About 1 cup of frozen mango chunks is equivalent to 1 medium fresh mango. Mango is a great source of vitamin C and potassium.

1 tablespoon toasted sesame oil

2 tablespoons minced fresh ginger

3 cloves garlic, peeled and minced

¼ cup soy sauce

3 tablespoons light brown sugar

1 teaspoon chili-garlic sauce

1 teaspoon vegetable oil

1 (2-pound) flank steak

1 teaspoon kosher salt, divided

1 teaspoon ground black pepper, divided

2 large mangoes, peeled, pitted, and diced

1 medium red bell pepper, seeded and diced

1 small shallot, peeled and minced

½ cup chopped fresh cilantro

1 tablespoon lime juice

SERVES 6

Per Serving

Calories	325
Fat	16g
Sodium	857mg
Carbohydrates	12g
Fiber	1g
Sugar	6g
Protein	33g

1 Heat sesame oil in a small saucepan over medium heat. Add ginger and garlic and sauté for 1 minute. Stir in soy sauce, brown sugar, and chili-garlic sauce. Cook, stirring frequently, until thickened and reduced, 4–5 minutes. Remove glaze from heat and set aside.

2 Preheat a gas or charcoal grill or set a grill pan over medium-high heat. Brush grill grates or grill pan with vegetable oil.

3 Season steak with ½ teaspoon each salt and black pepper and cook until desired doneness, 2–4 minutes per side. Transfer to a plate and brush with half the glaze. Cover with foil.

4 In a medium bowl, mix together mangoes, bell pepper, shallot, cilantro, lime juice, and remaining ½ teaspoon each salt and black pepper.

5 Slice steak against the grain and divide among six plates. Top with salsa and serve immediately.

Apricot-Stuffed Pork Tenderloin

SERVES 6

Per Serving

Calories	194
Fat	8g
Sodium	300mg
Carbohydrates	7g
Fiber	2g
Sugar	5g
Protein	24g

BE FOOD-SAFE!

Make sure you cook your pork until its internal temperature reaches 160°F to avoid exposure to potentially harmful food-borne bacteria.

You can swap in dried apricots instead of fresh. Just rehydrate them in a little red wine for about 15 minutes before using.

1 (1½-pound) pork tenderloin

1 small shallot, peeled and minced

3 cloves garlic, peeled and minced

6 medium apricots, pitted and sliced

½ cup chopped pecans

3 fresh sage leaves, chopped

¾ teaspoon kosher salt

½ teaspoon ground black pepper

1 Preheat oven to 375°F. Spray a roasting pan with a rack with non-stick cooking spray.

2 Place tenderloin on a cutting board. Make a lengthwise slice down the middle, being careful not to cut completely through. Open tenderloin like a book and flatten it with your hands.

3 Layer shallot, garlic, apricots, pecans, and sage over tenderloin and season with salt and pepper. Starting at one long side, carefully roll up tenderloin. Use butcher's twine to tie the roll at three or four places along the length.

4 Place tenderloin on the prepared rack and roast for 1–1½ hours until the internal temperature reaches 160°F. Let cool for 5 minutes before slicing. Serve warm.

Pork Medallions with Jalapeño Mustard

Jalapeños not only add a mild heat to dishes, but they're also a good source of vitamin A, vitamin C, and potassium.

¼ cup Dijon mustard

1 tablespoon honey

2 teaspoons minced garlic

2 tablespoons lemon juice

2 tablespoons minced jalapeño pepper

½ teaspoon garlic salt

6 tablespoons all-purpose flour

1 (1½-pound) pork tenderloin, trimmed and cut into 1" medallions

¼ teaspoon salt

½ teaspoon ground black pepper

3 tablespoons olive oil

1   Combine mustard, honey, garlic, lemon juice, jalapeño, and garlic salt in a small bowl and stir to combine. Set aside.

2   Place flour in a shallow bowl.

3   Season pork medallions with salt and pepper. Dredge pork in flour, shaking off excess.

4   Heat oil in a large nonstick skillet over medium-high heat. Add medallions and cook until both sides are golden brown, 6–7 minutes per side.

5   Add mustard mixture to the pan and stir to coat the medallions. Cook until pork is firm to the touch and no pink shows in the center, 2–3 minutes.

6   Remove the pan from heat, tent with foil, and let rest for 5 minutes. Stir to blend and serve hot.

SERVES 4

Per Serving

Calories	229
Fat	10g
Sodium	477mg
Carbohydrates	11g
Fiber	0g
Sugar	4g
Protein	24g

PUT DOWN THAT FORK!

Never use a fork to turn meats. It pierces the meat and allows the flavorful juices to escape. Use a spatula or tongs to gently turn or flip meats.

Shrimp Tostadas

SERVES 6

Per Serving

Calories	580
Fat	33g
Sodium	1,004mg
Carbohydrates	30g
Fiber	6g
Sugar	3g
Protein	41g

Chili powder is made from the dried and crushed powder of New Mexico chilies and ancho chilies. It contains iron and vitamin B_6 and acts as an anti-inflammatory agent in the body.

2 teaspoons chili powder

1 teaspoon ground cumin

1 teaspoon dried oregano

1 teaspoon garlic powder

1 teaspoon onion powder

1 teaspoon salt

2 pounds large shrimp, peeled and deveined

1 tablespoon olive oil

12 tostada shells

2 medium avocados, peeled, pitted, and sliced

2 cups shredded Mexican-style cheese

½ cup sour cream

1 head romaine lettuce, cored and shredded

2 medium tomatoes, cored and diced

1 Combine chili powder, cumin, oregano, garlic powder, onion powder, and salt in a large bowl. Add shrimp and toss to combine.
2 Heat oil in a large skillet over medium heat. Add shrimp and cook, turning once, until shrimp are cooked through, 2–3 minutes.
3 Top tostada shells with shrimp, avocado slices, cheese, sour cream, shredded lettuce, and tomatoes. Serve immediately.

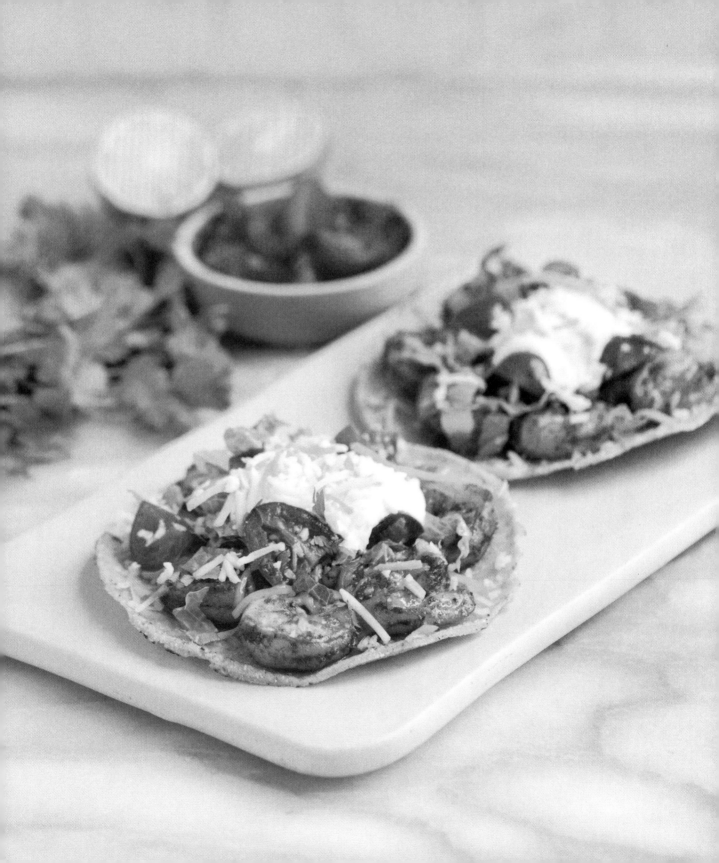

Walnut Shrimp

SERVES 6

Per Serving

Calories	590
Fat	30g
Sodium	517mg
Carbohydrates	41g
Fiber	2g
Sugar	12g
Protein	37g

Walnuts are a great source of alpha-linolenic acid, a plant-based omega-3 fatty acid that helps reduce inflammation in the body.

½ cup olive oil mayonnaise

¼ teaspoon garlic salt

1 teaspoon chili-garlic sauce

2 tablespoons honey

1 cup panko bread crumbs

2 large eggs

2 pounds large shrimp, peeled and deveined

¼ cup canola or vegetable oil

1 cup chopped candied walnuts

2 cups cooked long-grain white rice

1. In a large bowl, whisk together mayonnaise, garlic salt, chili-garlic sauce, and honey. Set aside.
2. Place panko in a shallow bowl. In another shallow bowl, lightly beat eggs with 1 tablespoon water. Dip shrimp into egg mixture, shake off excess, then dredge in panko. Place on a wire rack.
3. Heat oil in a large skillet over medium heat. Place breaded shrimp in the skillet in a single layer and cook for 2 minutes on each side, or until cooked through.
4. Transfer shrimp to the bowl with mayonnaise sauce and toss to coat. Top with walnuts and serve with rice.

Scallops Madras

Scallops are a great source of lean protein. They also contain selenium and zinc, two essential micronutrients that help reduce inflammation.

1 tablespoon ketchup

¼ cup low-fat coconut milk

¼ teaspoon kosher salt

⅛ teaspoon ground cayenne pepper

1 teaspoon curry powder

1 teaspoon garam masala

1 teaspoon minced garlic

2 tablespoons olive oil

1½ pounds sea scallops

1 tablespoon lemon juice

1. In a small bowl, whisk together ketchup, coconut milk, salt, and pepper. Set aside.
2. Combine curry powder, garam masala, garlic, and oil in a large bowl. Add scallops and toss to coat.
3. Heat a large nonstick skillet over medium-high heat. Add scallops and sear until almost cooked through, 1½–2 minutes, turning once. Stir in ketchup mixture. Continue to cook until sauce is reduced and scallops are opaque in the center and cooked through, 2–3 minutes. Stir in lemon juice. Serve hot.

SERVES 4

Per Serving

Calories	233
Fat	10g
Sodium	429mg
Carbohydrates	10g
Fiber	1g
Sugar	1g
Protein	26g

GETTING TO KNOW YOUR ANTI-INFLAMMATORY SPICES

Garam masala and curry powder are both spice blends common in South Asian cuisines. They're pungent, but not "hot." Together they contain a number of inflammation-fighting spices such as turmeric, fenugreek, black peppercorns, cloves, cinnamon, and cardamom.

Seared Scallops over Shaved Brussels Sprouts Salad

SERVES 4

Per Serving

Calories	573
Fat	23g
Sodium	972mg
Carbohydrates	47g
Fiber	13g
Sugar	24g
Protein	44g

To get the most even browning, make sure you allow scallops to come to room temperature and then pat them dry with a paper towel before searing.

2 cloves garlic, peeled and minced

¼ cup mayonnaise

2 tablespoons white wine vinegar

1 tablespoon Dijon mustard

1 tablespoon maple syrup

1 teaspoon dried basil

1½ teaspoons salt, divided

1 teaspoon ground black pepper, divided

2 pounds Brussels sprouts, trimmed and shredded

2 medium Honeycrisp apples, cored and diced

½ cup thinly sliced scallions

¼ cup pine nuts

2 pounds large sea scallops

2 tablespoons butter

1 In a large bowl, whisk together garlic, mayonnaise, vinegar, mustard, maple syrup, basil, ½ teaspoon salt, and ½ teaspoon pepper. Add Brussels sprouts, apples, scallions, and pine nuts. Toss to coat.

2 Pat scallops dry with paper towels and season with remaining 1 teaspoon salt and ½ teaspoon pepper.

3 Heat butter in a large skillet over medium-high heat. Place scallops in the skillet and cook for about 2 minutes on each side until a brown sear develops.

4 Divide Brussels sprouts mixture among four plates. Top with scallops and serve immediately.

Asian Salmon Patties

Salmon is a good source of omega-3 fats, and these patties make a great light lunch. Enjoy them over a lightly dressed salad or in a wrap with lettuce, tomato, and red onion.

1 large egg

1 tablespoon chopped fresh cilantro

1 teaspoon hoisin sauce

½ tablespoon mayonnaise

½ tablespoon chopped scallions

½ teaspoon minced fresh ginger

1 clove garlic, peeled and minced

1 teaspoon seasoned salt

½ teaspoon ground black pepper

¼ pound skinless salmon fillet, diced

3 tablespoons fresh bread crumbs

SERVES 1	
Per Serving	
Calories	317
Fat	19g
Sodium	1,142mg
Carbohydrates	8g
Fiber	0g
Sugar	2g
Protein	28g

1 In a large bowl, mix together egg, cilantro, hoisin sauce, mayonnaise, scallions, ginger, garlic, seasoned salt, and pepper. Add salmon and bread crumbs and lightly toss until blended. Form mixture into two patties.

2 Heat a small ungreased nonstick skillet over medium-high heat. Place salmon patties in skillet and cook until the undersides are golden, about 1½ minutes. Carefully flip and cook for 2 minutes more. Transfer patties to a plate and let rest for several minutes. Serve at room temperature.

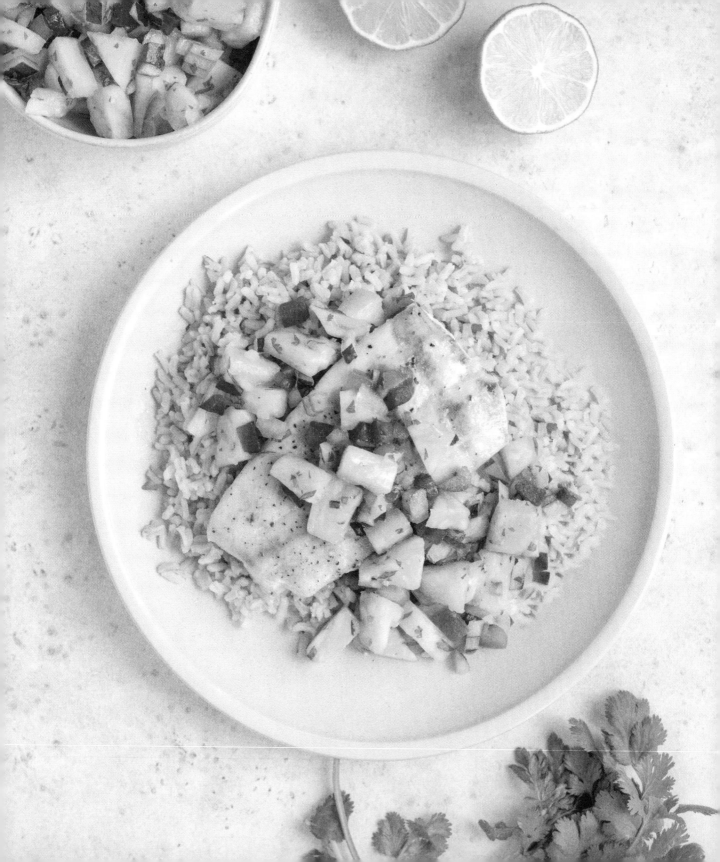

Grilled Mahi-Mahi with Pineapple Salsa

This salsa is also good on pork tenderloin. The fruit and vegetables add fiber, texture, and piquancy to simple grilled proteins. Serve this zesty dish with brown rice or quinoa.

1 cup diced pineapple

½ cup diced red onion

¼ cup minced green bell pepper

¼ cup minced red bell pepper

¼ bunch cilantro, stemmed and chopped

1 tablespoon white wine vinegar

¼ teaspoon hot pepper sauce

¼ teaspoon salt

2 pounds mahi-mahi or other firm-fleshed white fish

2 tablespoons olive oil

½ teaspoon ground black pepper

1. Combine pineapple, onion, bell peppers, and cilantro in a medium bowl. Add vinegar, hot sauce, and salt. Stir well and set aside.
2. Preheat a gas or charcoal grill.
3. Brush fish with oil and season with black pepper. Place on hot grill. Grill for 3–4 minutes per side until fish is opaque.
4. Serve fish with pineapple salsa.

SERVES 8

Per Serving

Calories	165
Fat	5g
Sodium	207mg
Carbohydrates	4g
Fiber	0g
Sugar	3g
Protein	26g

ANTI-INFLAMMATORY FRUITS

Pineapple contains an enzyme called bromelain. This enzyme may block pro-inflammatory substances that can speed up and worsen the inflammatory process. Extracts of bromelain may be a useful tool for fighting arthritis, but don't get too excited. It does not currently carry a health claim indicating its approval by the Food and Drug Administration. Still, until further research is completed, eat your pineapple!

Sweet Chili Salmon with Butternut Squash and Broccoli

This easy weeknight sheet pan meal comes together quickly with the help of premade sweet chili sauce, which pairs nicely with the salmon and vegetables.

1 small butternut squash, peeled, seeded, and diced

2 medium crowns broccoli, trimmed and cut into florets

1 tablespoon olive oil

4 tablespoons sweet chili sauce, divided

4 (8-ounce) salmon fillets

1 Preheat oven to 400° F. Line a large baking sheet with foil or a silicone baking mat.

2 In a large bowl, toss squash and broccoli with oil and 2 tablespoons chili sauce. Spread mixture onto the prepared baking sheet. Nestle fillets in between vegetables and brush with remaining sauce.

3 Bake for 15–20 minutes until salmon is cooked through and vegetables are fork-tender. Serve hot.

Grilled Tuna Steaks with Sautéed Leeks

Leeks have a sweet oniony flavor that's not as strong as that of yellow or red onions. Before cooking, be sure to rinse between all the layers of the leek to wash out any sand or grit.

1½ pounds tuna steaks (cut into 4-ounce portions)

1 tablespoon plus 1 teaspoon extra-virgin olive oil, divided

½ teaspoon salt

½ teaspoon ground black pepper

3 large leeks (white and light green parts only), thinly sliced

1 tablespoon lemon juice

1 tablespoon honey

1 Preheat a gas or charcoal grill.

2 Brush tuna with 1 tablespoon oil and season with salt and pepper. Place tuna on grill; cook for 3 minutes. Shift tuna steaks to form an *X*-shaped grill pattern; cook 3 minutes more.

3 Turn steaks over and grill 3 minutes more, then change position again to create an *X* grill pattern. Cook 1–3 minutes more to desired doneness. Remove from grill and keep warm.

4 Heat remaining 1 teaspoon oil in a medium skillet over medium heat. Sauté leeks 3–4 minutes until wilted. Remove from heat and add lemon juice and honey. Serve tuna steaks with a spoonful of leek mixture on top.

SERVES 6

Per Serving

Calories	134
Fat	3g
Sodium	194mg
Carbohydrates	3g
Fiber	1g
Sugar	3g
Protein	24g

TERRIFIC TUNA

Tuna is truly a nutrient-dense food. This omega-3 fatty acid–rich fish has anti-inflammation written all over it, with heaps of other valuable disease-fighting nutrients as well. Try to eat fish at least twice a week to reap the significant health benefits.

Grilled Red Snapper with Polenta

SERVES 6

Per Serving

Calories	369
Fat	10g
Sodium	643mg
Carbohydrates	33g
Fiber	1g
Sugar	1g
Protein	37g

SNAPPER IS SUPER

Snapper is high in protein and low in saturated fat while providing 15 percent of the daily value for omega-3 fatty acids in a 4-ounce serving. It's also a good source of potassium, vitamin A, and selenium.

Try out different types of fish with this recipe. Grouper, catfish, haddock, or cod would all work well with this combination of flavors. If you can't find Manchego cheese, you can substitute Monterey jack, mozzarella, or Cheddar cheese.

3 teaspoons olive oil, divided

½ small serrano pepper, seeded and diced

1 quart low-sodium seafood or chicken stock

1½ cups cornmeal

3 ounces grated Manchego cheese

1½ pounds red snapper (cut into 4-ounce portions)

½ teaspoon salt

½ teaspoon ground black pepper

1 tablespoon apple cider vinegar

1. Heat 2 teaspoons oil in a large saucepan or Dutch oven over medium heat. Sauté serrano pepper for 1 minute, then add stock and bring to a boil.
2. Whisk in cornmeal slowly. Cook for 20–30 minutes, stirring frequently, until all liquid has been absorbed and polenta is thickened. Remove from heat and stir in cheese. Set aside and keep warm.
3. Preheat a gas or charcoal grill.
4. Brush fish with remaining 1 teaspoon oil and season with salt and black pepper. Grill fillets for 3–5 minutes on each side until fish flakes easily with a fork.
5. Drizzle fish with vinegar and serve over polenta.

CHAPTER 12

Dessert

Strawberry Parfait

SERVES 4

Per Serving

Calories	156
Fat	7g
Sodium	2mg
Carbohydrates	22g
Fiber	10g
Sugar	12g
Protein	1g

Not only do mint leaves add a delicious flavor to desserts, but they are also a strong anti-inflammatory herb and can aid in digestion.

1 cup sliced strawberries

1½ cups nondairy whipped topping, thawed

½ cup sugar-free strawberry preserves

4 whole strawberries

4 small mint leaves

1 Divide sliced strawberries equally among four chilled martini glasses or ramekins.

2 Combine whipped topping with the preserves in a medium bowl and stir until evenly blended. Dollop mixture on top of strawberries or use a piping bag to top each with a rosette.

3 Garnish each serving with a whole strawberry and a mint leaf.

Crunchy Peach Parfait

SERVES 1

Per Serving

Calories	693
Fat	27g
Sodium	153mg
Carbohydrates	77g
Fiber	1g
Sugar	51g
Protein	35g

If you can't find fresh peaches, you can easily substitute frozen peach chunks. Simply let them thaw before adding to the parfait.

1 cup low-fat plain Greek yogurt

½ teaspoon vanilla extract

1 tablespoon maple syrup

1 cup sliced fresh peaches

½ cup granola

6 walnut halves, roughly chopped

1 In a small bowl, stir together yogurt, vanilla, and maple syrup.

2 In a tall glass or glass bowl, begin with a layer of yogurt mixture, then peaches, and finally granola. Repeat layering to fill glass.

3 Sprinkle walnuts on top and serve immediately.

Roasted Peaches with Yogurt

Peaches are in season during the summer months. Buy them before they're fully ripe and wait until they give a little when lightly pressed. They'll be perfect for roasting.

2 large ripe peaches, halved and pitted

1 tablespoon butter, cut into 4 pieces

4 teaspoons light brown sugar

½ teaspoon ground cinnamon

2 cups whole-fat plain Greek yogurt

½ teaspoon vanilla extract

1 teaspoon honey

½ cup chopped roasted pecans

1 Preheat oven to 350°F.

2 Place peach halves in a medium ungreased baking dish and top with butter, brown sugar, and cinnamon. Bake for 30–40 minutes until peaches can be pierced easily with a knife.

3 In a medium bowl, whisk together yogurt, vanilla, and honey.

4 Divide peach halves among four dessert plates and top with yogurt mixture and pecans. Serve immediately.

SERVES 4

Per Serving

Calories	259
Fat	12g
Sodium	66mg
Carbohydrates	25g
Fiber	1g
Sugar	18g
Protein	13g

WORKING WITH YOGURT

Mixing yogurt in a blender can cause it to break down and become liquefied. Instead, either whisk it gently or fold the yogurt into the mixture when incorporating it into most recipes.

Strawberry Sorbet

SORBET OR SHERBET?

Sherbet (not "sherbert," as it's often mispronounced) includes milk. It's like a watery ice cream. Sorbet contains no milk or other dairy products. Sorbets, Italian ices, and granitas are all related, giving you a great fruity chill-down on a hot day or after an evening meal. If they are made with puréed ingredients, they will have less fiber, but you can always serve them with berries, cut-up peaches, or whatever is in season.

Strawberries are a good source of vitamin C and polyphenols, plant chemicals that have great anti-inflammatory effects.

2 quarts strawberries, hulled

¾ cup sugar

¼ cup lemon juice

1 Purée strawberries in a blender or food processor until smooth. Add sugar and lemon juice and pulse to combine. Transfer purée to a covered container and refrigerate for at least 2 hours.

2 Freeze in an ice cream maker according to manufacturer's instructions, then transfer to a covered container and freeze for 2–3 hours until firm.

3 If you don't have an ice cream machine, transfer sorbet mixture to a freezer-safe bowl or container. Cover tightly with plastic wrap, foil, or an airtight cover. Freeze for 2 hours. Remove from freezer and beat with a hand mixer to break up ice crystals. Cover and return to freezer. Freeze for 2 hours more. Remove from freezer and beat again with a hand mixer. Sorbet should be thick but too soft to scoop. Freeze for 2–3 hours until firm.

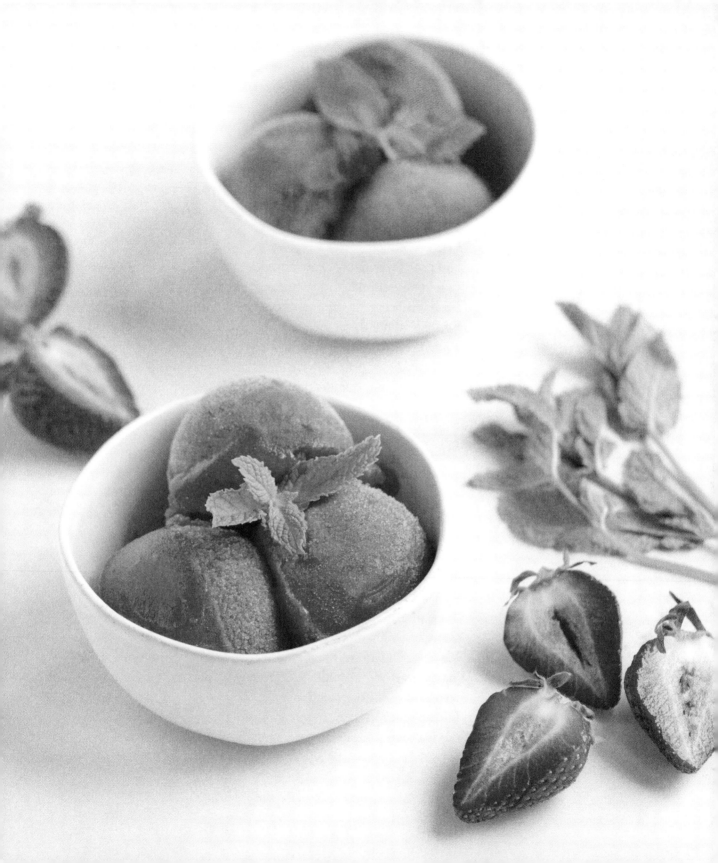

Caramelized Pears with Toasted Almonds

SERVES 4	
Per Serving	
Calories	99
Fat	3g
Sodium	12mg
Carbohydrates	14g
Fiber	2g
Sugar	8g
Protein	4g

Use pears that are ripe but still firm; overly ripe pears will cook too quickly.

3 large pears, ripe but firm, quartered, cored, and thinly sliced

1 tablespoon light brown sugar

2 tablespoons sliced almonds

½ cup low-fat vanilla Greek yogurt

4 small mint leaves

1 Preheat broiler.

2 Fan pear slices in concentric circles in a shallow ungreased oven-proof pan. Sprinkle brown sugar over pears.

3 Broil until sugar is caramelized, but not burned, about 5 minutes. Sprinkle almonds on top and broil for 1 minute more or until golden.

4 To serve, divide pears among four serving plates. Top each with a spoonful of yogurt and garnish with mint leaves. Serve immediately.

Grilled Pineapple with Whipped Cream

SERVES 4	
Per Serving	
Calories	352
Fat	20g
Sodium	43mg
Carbohydrates	42g
Fiber	3g
Sugar	25g
Protein	1g

Pineapple contains the plant enzyme bromelain, which can help reduce chronic inflammation in the body.

1 medium pineapple, peeled, cored, and sliced into rings

¼ cup light brown sugar

1 teaspoon ground cinnamon

1 cup whipped heavy cream

4 maraschino cherries

1 Place pineapple rings in a large bowl and sprinkle with brown sugar and cinnamon. Toss to coat.

2 Place a grill pan over medium heat and spray with nonstick cooking spray. Add pineapple slices and cook until soft and caramelized, 3–4 minutes per side.

3 Divide pineapple rings among four dessert plates. Top each serving with whipped cream and a cherry. Serve immediately.

Raspberry Rhubarb Crisp

Rhubarb is rich in anthocyanins, a plant pigment that gives it its red color and is a potent antioxidant. The only edible part of the plant is the vibrant pink stem.

6 cups chopped rhubarb stalks, red part only

1¾ cups all-purpose flour, divided

1¼ cups granulated sugar, divided

2 cups raspberries

1 cup almond meal

¼ cup old-fashioned rolled oats

½ cup light brown sugar

1 teaspoon ground cinnamon

½ teaspoon salt

¾ cup unsalted butter, cut into chunks

1 Preheat oven to 350°F.

2 In a large bowl, toss rhubarb with ¼ cup flour and 1 cup granulated sugar. Add raspberries and toss gently. Transfer mixture to a 9" × 11" ungreased baking dish. Set aside.

3 In a medium bowl, combine remaining 1½ cups flour and ¼ cup granulated sugar, almond meal, oats, brown sugar, cinnamon, and salt. Add butter chunks and mix to a sandy consistency with an electric mixer.

4 Cover raspberry mixture evenly with almond mixture and bake for 1 hour or until the juices start to bubble up and thicken.

5 Remove crisp from oven and cut around the sides to loosen. Cool for 20 minutes, then cut into squares and serve warm.

SERVES 8

Per Serving

Calories	501
Fat	20g
Sodium	166mg
Carbohydrates	72g
Fiber	6g
Sugar	35g
Protein	8g

LIGHT VS. DARK BROWN SUGAR

The difference between light and dark brown sugar is simply the amount of molasses added. Dark brown sugar will provide a more robust flavor and darker result.

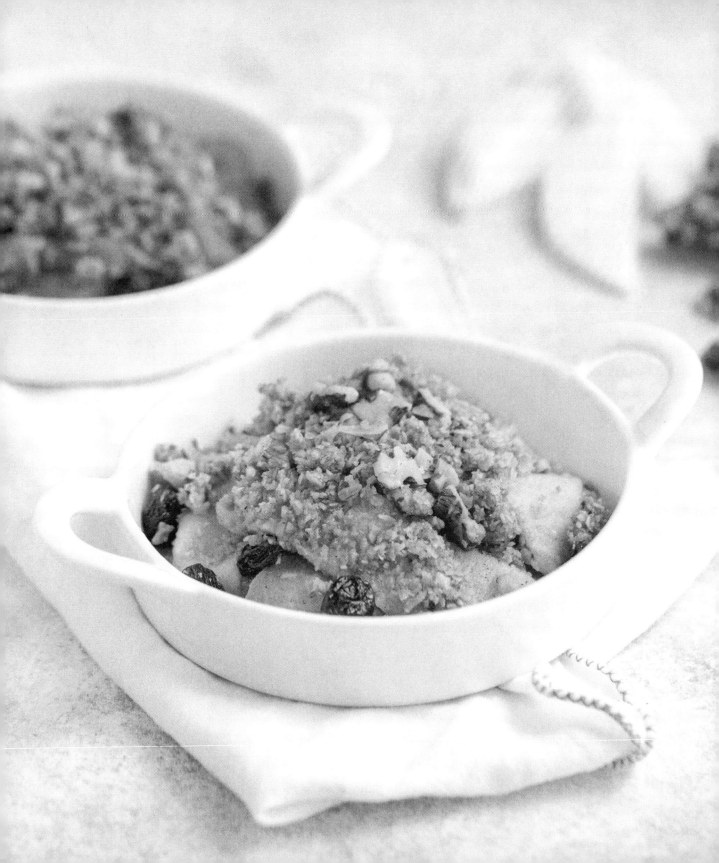

Quick Apple Crisp

There is nothing like the taste of maple syrup, apples, and cinnamon heated together and baked. Apple crisp is an American classic the whole family will enjoy. Serve warm with a scoop of vanilla ice cream or a spoonful of Greek yogurt.

5 large apples, peeled, cored, and sliced

½ cup raisins

½ cup apple juice

3 tablespoons lemon juice

1 teaspoon ground cinnamon

¼ cup plus ⅔ cup maple syrup, divided

2 cups old-fashioned rolled oats

½ cup chopped walnuts

¼ teaspoon salt

1 teaspoon vanilla extract

⅓ cup canola oil

1. Preheat oven to 350°F.
2. Layer apples with raisins in a 9" × 12" ungreased baking dish.
3. In a small bowl, whisk together apple juice, lemon juice, cinnamon, and ¼ cup maple syrup; pour over apples and raisins.
4. Process oats in a food processor until they reach a flour consistency. Add walnuts and salt; pulse to lightly chop. Pour the mixture into a large bowl.
5. In a small bowl, whisk together vanilla, oil, and remaining ⅔ cup maple syrup. Pour over oat mixture and stir to combine.
6. Spoon oat mixture over apple mixture. Bake for 30 minutes or until apples are tender and topping is golden brown.
7. Allow to cool slightly before serving.

SERVES 8

Per Serving

Calories	403
Fat	16g
Sodium	84mg
Carbohydrates	59g
Fiber	6g
Sugar	43g
Protein	5g

MAPLE SYRUP

Maple syrup is made from the sap of the sugar, black, or red maple tree. The tree is first tapped (pierced), which allows the sap to run out freely. The clear, tasteless sap is then boiled down to evaporate the water, giving it the characteristic maple flavor and amber color, with a sugar content of 60 percent.

Nectarine Cherry Tart with Oat Crumble Topping

Nectarines are actually a type of peach, but without the fuzzy outer skin. They are high in vitamin C and fiber.

2 large ripe nectarines, pitted and thinly sliced

2 cups pitted cherries

3 tablespoons instant tapioca

1 cup firmly packed light brown sugar, divided

1 tablespoon cold butter, diced

1 teaspoon vanilla extract

1 (9") deep-dish pie crust

1 cup old-fashioned rolled oats

1 cup toasted walnut pieces

3 tablespoons all-purpose flour

¼ cup butter, softened

1. Preheat oven to 350°F.
2. In a large bowl, toss together nectarine slices and cherries, then stir in tapioca and ½ cup brown sugar. Add cold butter and vanilla and stir. Spoon mixture into pie crust.
3. In a medium bowl, combine oats, walnuts, remaining ½ cup brown sugar, flour, and softened butter and mix until crumbly. Sprinkle over filling and press down.
4. Bake until topping is brown, about 30 minutes. Serve warm.

Blackberry Cobbler

This fruit cobbler can also be made using raspberries, blueberries, cherries, or a mix of fruits. The berry juice soaks into the biscuits, giving them great flavor. The whole-wheat flour in the biscuits provides protein and fiber.

1 recipe Whole-Wheat Biscuits (see recipe in this chapter), unbaked

8 cups blackberries

¼ cup all-purpose flour

¾ cup sugar

¼ cup heavy cream

SERVES 8	
Per Serving	
Calories	463
Fat	15g
Sodium	481mg
Carbohydrates	73g
Fiber	12g
Sugar	30g
Protein	9g

1 Preheat oven to 350°F.

2 Roll Whole-Wheat Biscuits dough on a floured surface to 1" thickness. Cut circles with a 2" or 3" round cookie cutter or drinking glass. Place rounds on a large ungreased baking sheet and set aside.

3 In a large bowl, toss together blackberries, flour, and sugar, then transfer to an ungreased 9" × 11" baking dish.

4 Bake for 25 minutes, remove from oven, and place unbaked biscuits on top of the hot berries. Brush biscuit tops with cream and return cobbler to the oven to bake for another 25 minutes.

5 Serve warm.

Whole-Wheat Biscuits

SERVES 8

Per Serving

Calories	287
Fat	12g
Sodium	477mg
Carbohydrates	38g
Fiber	4g
Sugar	4g
Protein	7g

These quick, not-too-sweet biscuits can be made in just under 30 minutes and can be used in desserts like Blackberry Cobbler (see recipe in this chapter) or strawberry shortcake.

1½ cups all-purpose flour

1½ cups whole-wheat flour

4½ teaspoons baking powder

1½ teaspoons salt

1 tablespoon sugar

6 tablespoons cold butter, cut into small pieces

1¼ cups buttermilk

1 Preheat oven to 400°F.

2 Combine flours, baking powder, salt, and sugar in a large bowl.

3 Add butter to flour mixture and mix in with a pastry cutter or your fingers until the mixture resembles small pebbles. Add buttermilk and mix with a wooden spoon to form the dough.

4 Roll dough on a floured surface to 1" thickness. Cut circles with a 2" or 3" round cookie cutter or drinking glass. Place rounds on a large ungreased baking sheet and bake for 12 minutes.

5 Serve warm or at room temperature.

Sesame Seed Cookies

These elegant, delicate cookies are a type of lace cookie, and they're full of delicious and fiber-rich sesame seeds. The seeds also add a touch of protein.

4½ teaspoons honey

1½ tablespoons butter

½ cup confectioners' sugar

1 tablespoon water

½ cup sesame seeds

⅛ teaspoon salt

2 tablespoons all-purpose flour

1 In a medium saucepan over medium heat, stir together honey, butter, sugar, and water and bring to a boil. Boil for 1 minute, then remove from heat.

2 Stir in sesame seeds, salt, and flour. Set aside to cool for 20 minutes.

3 Preheat oven to 350°F. Line two large baking sheets with parchment paper.

4 Roll cookie dough into 1" balls and place them 4" apart on the prepared baking sheets.

5 Bake for 8 minutes. Transfer cookies to a wire rack to cool.

MAKES 15 COOKIES

Per Serving (1 cookie)

Calories	63
Fat	3g
Sodium	31mg
Carbohydrates	8g
Fiber	1g
Sugar	6g
Protein	1g

Oatmeal Raisin Chewies

Per Serving (1 cookie)

Calories	254
Fat	9g
Sodium	41mg
Carbohydrates	39g
Fiber	4g
Sugar	18g
Protein	4g

CHOOSING VANILLA EXTRACT

Read the label carefully when choosing vanilla extract. Be sure it says "100% vanilla extract," and not "imitation vanilla." Some of the compounds found in real vanilla extract have antioxidant effects.

Spelt is an ancient grain that has a higher protein content than white flour.

2 tablespoons canola oil, divided

1½ cups old-fashioned rolled oats

¾ cup spelt flour

⅛ teaspoon salt

½ cup chopped walnuts

½ cup raisins

1 teaspoon ground cinnamon

⅓ cup agave or maple syrup

½ teaspoon vanilla extract

1 cup cold water

1 Preheat oven to 375°F. Brush two baking sheets with ½ tablespoon oil.

2 In a large bowl, mix oats, flour, salt, walnuts, raisins, and cinnamon. Add remaining 1½ tablespoons oil slowly, making sure to coat oats well with oil.

3 Slowly stir in syrup and vanilla. Add water; mix until batter becomes thick.

4 Using a tablespoon, spoon batter onto the prepared baking sheets. Pat down each spoonful into a patty about 2" across and ¼" thick. Place patties ½" apart. The cookies will not spread.

5 Bake for 25 minutes or until golden brown.

6 Cool cookies slightly before transferring to a wire rack. Cool completely before serving.

Peanut Butter Chocolate Chip Cookies

Peanut butter contains oleic acid, a heart-healthy fat that can help reduce blood pressure and blood sugar.

½ cup granulated sugar

½ cup packed brown sugar

½ cup creamy natural peanut butter

½ cup butter, softened

1 large egg

1¼ cups all-purpose flour

¾ teaspoon baking soda

½ teaspoon baking powder

¼ teaspoon salt

1 cup semisweet chocolate chips

1 In a large bowl, beat together granulated sugar, brown sugar, peanut butter, butter, and egg for 1 minute or until light and creamy. In a medium bowl, mix together flour, baking soda, baking powder, and salt. Add flour mixture to peanut butter mixture, stirring well to combine into a smooth dough. Fold in chocolate chips. Cover and refrigerate for 2 hours.

2 Preheat oven to 375°F. Line two large baking sheets with parchment paper.

3 Scoop teaspoonfuls of dough and roll into balls. Place balls on the prepared baking sheets, leaving a 1" space between each cookie. Flatten balls in crisscross patterns with a fork.

4 Bake for 8–10 minutes until very lightly browned. Let cool on baking sheets for 5 minutes, then transfer to a wire rack to cool completely.

MAKES 30 COOKIES

Per Serving (1 cookie)

Calories	132
Fat	7g
Sodium	47mg
Carbohydrates	15g
Fiber	1g
Sugar	11g
Protein	2g

CHILLING COOKIE DOUGH

Chilling dough before baking cookies helps to solidify the fat. As the cookies bake, the fat melts more slowly than room-temperature fat, so the cookies spread less.

Apricot Chocolate Chip Squares

SERVES 18

Per Serving

Calories	383
Fat	20g
Sodium	78mg
Carbohydrates	45g
Fiber	2g
Sugar	19g
Protein	6g

These easy-to-make cookies feature sweet fruit, rich chocolate, and the crunch of granola and cashews. Pack these instead of trail mix when you go camping or hiking.

1 cup unsalted butter, softened

¾ cup light brown sugar

¾ cup granulated sugar

3 large eggs or ¾ cup egg substitute

1 teaspoon vanilla extract

1¼ cups all-purpose flour

1 cup whole-wheat flour

½ teaspoon salt

2 teaspoons baking soda

1 cup semisweet chocolate chips

1 cup chopped dried apricots

2 cups granola

1 cup chopped cashews

1 Preheat oven to 375°F. Line a 15½" × 10½" × 1" baking sheet with foil.

2 In a large bowl, cream butter and sugars with an electric mixer until fluffy.

3 Add eggs and vanilla and combine well. Scrape the sides of the bowl.

4 Mix flours, salt, and baking soda together in a medium bowl. Add flour mixture to the butter mixture, stirring well to combine into a smooth dough. Fold in chocolate chips, dried apricots, granola, and cashews.

5 Press dough into prepared pan and bake for 20 minutes. Cool on a rack for at least 1 hour. Cut into squares before serving.

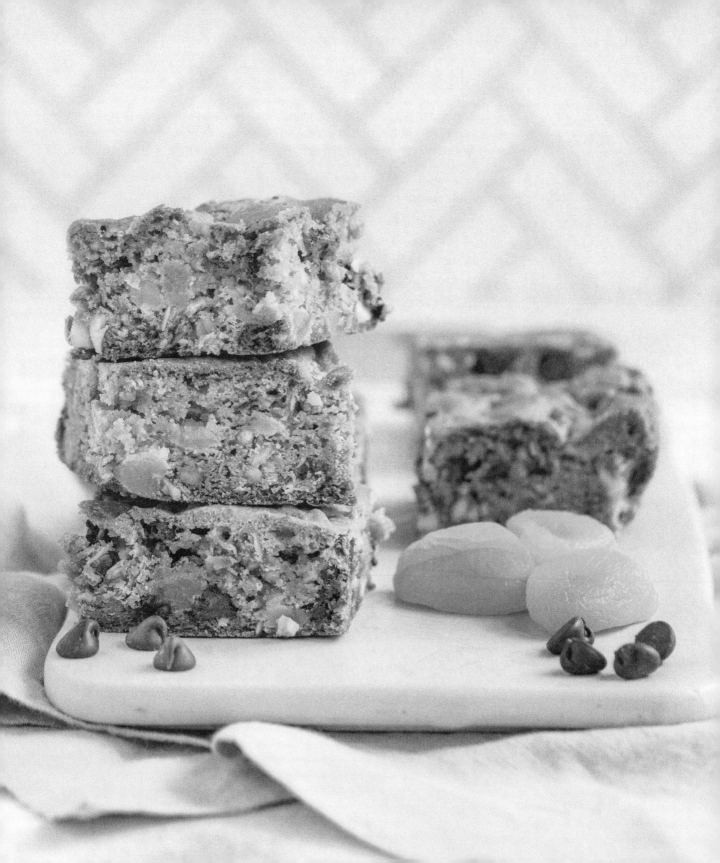

Almond Cookies

MAKES 24 COOKIES

Per Serving (1 cookie)

Calories	28
Fat	0g
Sodium	7mg
Carbohydrates	6g
Fiber	0g
Sugar	4g
Protein	1g

SWEET TOOTH

Adding sweet spices such as cinnamon, nutmeg, or cardamom will enhance the perception of sweetness in your desserts, even if they don't contain a lot of sugar.

Almond meal is made from raw, unpeeled almonds and is rich in vitamin E. These cookies should be stored in an airtight container. To restore their original crisp texture, heat them in a 200°F oven for 1–2 minutes.

7 tablespoons sugar

3 large egg whites, at room temperature

½ cup almond meal

⅓ cup cake flour

1 teaspoon Cointreau liqueur

¼ teaspoon vanilla extract

1. Preheat oven to 425°F. Line two large baking sheets with parchment paper.
2. In a large bowl, whisk sugar and egg whites until whites are frothy and sugar substitute is dissolved. Add remaining ingredients and whisk until smooth.
3. Place rounded teaspoons of dough on the prepared baking sheets, leaving a 1" space between each cookie.
4. Bake for 5–6 minutes until the edges turn golden. Remove from oven and transfer cookies to a wire rack. Let cool completely.

Energy Oat Bars

Rice syrup is a thick, mild sweetener that helps bind the bars together. If you want a sweeter bar, substitute ½ cup agave or maple syrup or honey.

¾ cup rice syrup

1½ cups almond butter

1 teaspoon vanilla extract

½ cup flaxseed meal

⅓ cup unsweetened coconut

½ cup old-fashioned rolled oats

⅓ cup raisins

⅓ cup chopped walnuts

1 In a large heavy saucepan, heat rice syrup over low heat until thin and runny, about 2 minutes. Add almond butter and vanilla; stir well.

2 Remove from heat. Stir in remaining ingredients; mix well.

3 Spoon mixture into an ungreased 8" × 8" baking pan and spread evenly. Score the dough into 20 pieces.

4 Cover and refrigerate for at least 2 hours. Following the scored lines, cut into 20 pieces and remove from pan. Keep refrigerated in a covered container for up to 1 week.

SERVES 20

Per Serving

Calories	196
Fat	13g
Sodium	5mg
Carbohydrates	15g
Fiber	3g
Sugar	9g
Protein	5g

Raspberry Almond Turnovers

PUFF PASTRY

Unfortunately, you can't buy whole-grain puff pastry, but you can fill it with fruit and nuts for wonderful turnovers. Wheat germ is also an excellent source of vitamins and fiber, and can be added to everything from meatloaf to pancake batter.

Delicious for breakfast but also a good dessert or snack, these turnovers are naturally high in fiber. Make a double batch and freeze them in individual portions to enjoy later in the week.

1 cup sliced almonds, divided

1 sheet puff pastry, thawed in the refrigerator

1 large egg white, lightly beaten, divided

4 teaspoons almond paste

1 cup frozen raspberries

4 teaspoons granulated sugar

2 teaspoons cornstarch

1 tablespoon wheat germ

2 tablespoons confectioners' sugar

1. Preheat oven to 400°F. Grind ½ cup almonds in a food processor. Set aside.
2. Roll puff pastry into an 11" × 11" square on a floured surface. Cut the square into four smaller squares. Brush some egg white on the pastry squares.
3. Put 1 teaspoon almond paste in the middle of each square, layer ¼ cup raspberries on top of each, then sprinkle ground almonds, granulated sugar, cornstarch, and wheat germ over berries.
4. Fold each square over to make a triangle to encase the filling. Press down on the outer edges with your fingers or a fork to seal.
5. Brush remaining egg white on top of turnovers and sprinkle them with confectioners' sugar and remaining ½ cup sliced almonds.
6. Bake for 10 minutes, then reduce oven temperature to 350°F and continue baking for 10–15 minutes longer, until pastry is lightly browned and flaky. Let cool before serving.

Dark Chocolate Cherry Cake with Ganache

This easy chocolate cake is moist and fudgy. Using chocolate cake mix means you can have an impressive dessert made in no time.

1 (15.25-ounce) package dark chocolate cake mix

1 (21-ounce) can cherry pie filling

1 teaspoon almond extract

2 large eggs

8 ounces bittersweet dark chocolate baking bars, finely chopped

1 cup heavy cream

8 maraschino cherries

1 Preheat oven to 350°F. Grease an 8" × 8" baking pan.

2 In a large bowl, combine cake mix, pie filling, almond extract, and eggs. Pour into the prepared baking pan. Bake for 30 minutes or until a toothpick inserted in the center comes out clean. Let the cake cool in the pan for 5 minutes, then transfer to a wire rack. Cool for at least 1 hour.

3 Place chocolate in a medium heatproof bowl. Heat cream in a small saucepan over medium heat, stirring constantly, until it simmers. Pour hot cream over chocolate, wait 2 minutes, then slowly stir until chocolate is melted and combined with cream. Let cool for 2 hours, stirring every 30 minutes.

4 Once it is cool and thickened, beat chocolate mixture with an electric mixer using a whisk attachment until light and fluffy, 4–5 minutes.

5 Spread ganache over cooled cake. Garnish with maraschino cherries and serve.

SERVES 8

Per Serving

Calories	590
Fat	27g
Sodium	391mg
Carbohydrates	80g
Fiber	5g
Sugar	39g
Protein	6g

DARK CHOCOLATE BENEFITS

Dark chocolate is lower in sugar than milk chocolate, and contains more flavonoids, iron, magnesium, and zinc.

Chocolate Peanut Butter Smoothie

SERVES 2	
Per Serving	
Calories	190
Fat	9g
Sodium	245mg
Carbohydrates	21g
Fiber	4g
Sugar	11g
Protein	6g

This smoothie is perfect for when you need a chocolate fix. It's also great for getting a little calcium and some healthy fats into your diet.

2 cups almond or oat milk

1 large banana, peeled, sliced, and frozen

2 tablespoons peanut butter

1 tablespoon cocoa powder

Combine ingredients in a blender; purée until smooth. Divide between two glasses; serve immediately.

Sample Meal Plans

Week 1				
	Breakfast	**Snack**	**Lunch**	**Dinner**
Monday	Coconut Turmeric Smoothie Bowls (Chapter 2)	Curry Cayenne Peanuts (Chapter 3)	Minestrone (Chapter 4)	Crispy Sweet Chili Tofu Sticks with Broccoli Slaw (Chapter 9)
Tuesday	Strawberry Banana Smoothie (Chapter 2)	Cottage cheese and berries	Vegan Niçoise Salad Bowls (Chapter 6)	Lentil Sloppy Joes (Chapter 10) with Citrus-Steamed Carrots (Chapter 5)
Wednesday	Peach Yogurt Smoothie (Chapter 2)	Peanut butter and apple slices	Quinoa Black Bean Salad (Chapter 6)	Creamy Avocado Fettuccine (Chapter 7)
Thursday	Morning Sunshine Smoothie (Chapter 2)	Carrot sticks and hummus	Black Bean Chili (Chapter 4)	Soy-Glazed Steak with Mango Salsa (Chapter 11)
Friday	Raisin Bran Muffins (Chapter 2)	Spicy Roasted Chickpeas (Chapter 3)	Quinoa Parsley Tabbouleh (Chapter 7)	Spicy Chicken Burgers (Chapter 11) with Grilled Vegetable Kebabs (Chapter 5)
Saturday	Vegan Eggs Benedict with Smoky Tempeh Bacon (Chapter 2)	Greek yogurt with granola	Two-Bean Chili Wraps (Chapter 8)	Seared Scallops over Shaved Brussels Sprouts Salad (Chapter 11)
Sunday	Crepes with Blueberry Sauce (Chapter 2)	Hard-cooked eggs and berries	Vegan BLTs with Tempeh Bacon (Chapter 8)	Creamy Chipotle Tempeh with Cilantro Lime Rice (Chapter 9)

Week 2

	Breakfast	Snack	Lunch	Dinner
Monday	Fresh Fruit Kebabs with Vanilla Yogurt Sauce (Chapter 2)	Pretzels with chocolate hummus	Thai Coconut Tofu Soup (Chapter 4)	Pasta e Ceci (Chapter 7)
Tuesday	Strawberry Banana Smoothie (Chapter 2)	Apple and Cheddar cheese slices	Creamy Dill Chickpea Salad Sandwiches (Chapter 8)	Vegan Meatloaf Cups (Chapter 9) with mashed potatoes and green beans
Wednesday	Savory Steel-Cut Oatmeal with Avocado and Fried Eggs (Chapter 2)	Peanut butter and blueberry preserve sandwich on whole-wheat bread	Curried Red Lentils and Tomatoes (Chapter 10)	Pita Pizzas with Roasted Garlic White Sauce (Chapter 8)
Thursday	Spinach, Mushroom, and Tomato Tofu Scramble (Chapter 2)	Raisin Bran Muffins (Chapter 2)	Creamy Wild Rice Soup (Chapter 4)	Lasagna Florentine (Chapter 7)
Friday	Blueberry Almond Breakfast Bars (Chapter 2)	Pistachios with fresh berries	White Bean Macaroni and Cheeze (Chapter 10)	Spicy Thai Basil Tofu (Chapter 9)
Saturday	Edamame Omelet (Chapter 2)	Energy Oat Bars (Chapter 12)	Cheezy Vegan Beef Burritos (Chapter 8)	Falafel Sandwiches (Chapter 8)
Sunday	Apple Bread (Chapter 2)	Apricot Chocolate Chip Squares (Chapter 12)	Vegan BLTs with Tempeh Bacon (Chapter 8)	Wild Rice Stir-Fry with Snow Peas and Broccolini (Chapter 7)

STANDARD US/METRIC MEASUREMENT CONVERSIONS

VOLUME CONVERSIONS

US Volume Measure	Metric Equivalent
⅛ teaspoon	0.5 milliliter
¼ teaspoon	1 milliliter
½ teaspoon	2 milliliters
1 teaspoon	5 milliliters
½ tablespoon	7 milliliters
1 tablespoon (3 teaspoons)	15 milliliters
2 tablespoons (1 fluid ounce)	30 milliliters
¼ cup (4 tablespoons)	60 milliliters
⅓ cup	90 milliliters
½ cup (4 fluid ounces)	125 milliliters
⅔ cup	160 milliliters
¾ cup (6 fluid ounces)	180 milliliters
1 cup (16 tablespoons)	250 milliliters
1 pint (2 cups)	500 milliliters
1 quart (4 cups)	1 liter (about)

WEIGHT CONVERSIONS

US Weight Measure	Metric Equivalent
½ ounce	15 grams
1 ounce	30 grams
2 ounces	60 grams
3 ounces	85 grams
¼ pound (4 ounces)	115 grams
½ pound (8 ounces)	225 grams
¾ pound (12 ounces)	340 grams
1 pound (16 ounces)	454 grams

OVEN TEMPERATURE CONVERSIONS

Degrees Fahrenheit	Degrees Celsius
200 degrees F	95 degrees C
250 degrees F	120 degrees C
275 degrees F	135 degrees C
300 degrees F	150 degrees C
325 degrees F	160 degrees C
350 degrees F	180 degrees C
375 degrees F	190 degrees C
400 degrees F	205 degrees C
425 degrees F	220 degrees C
450 degrees F	230 degrees C

BAKING PAN SIZES

American	Metric
8 × 1½ inch round baking pan	20 × 4 cm cake tin
9 × 1½ inch round baking pan	23 × 3.5 cm cake tin
11 × 7 × 1½ inch baking pan	28 × 18 × 4 cm baking tin
13 × 9 × 2 inch baking pan	30 × 20 × 5 cm baking tin
2 quart rectangular baking dish	30 × 20 × 3 cm baking tin
15 × 10 × 2 inch baking pan	30 × 25 × 2 cm baking tin (Swiss roll tin)
9 inch pie plate	22 × 4 or 23 × 4 cm pie plate
7 or 8 inch springform pan	18 or 20 cm springform or loose bottom cake tin
9 × 5 × 3 inch loaf pan	23 × 13 × 7 cm or 2 lb narrow loaf or pate tin
1½ quart casserole	1.5 liter casserole
2 quart casserole	2 liter casserole

Index

Healthy and delicious Mediterranean recipes the whole family will love!

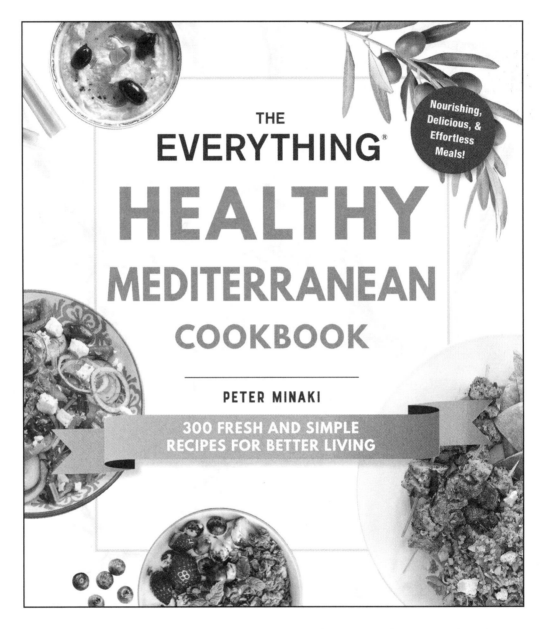

THE
EVERYTHING®
HEALTHY
MEDITERRANEAN
COOKBOOK

PETER MINAKI

300 FRESH AND SIMPLE RECIPES FOR BETTER LIVING

Nourishing, Delicious, & Effortless Meals!

PICK UP OR DOWNLOAD YOUR COPY TODAY!

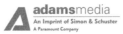

adamsmedia
An Imprint of Simon & Schuster
A Paramount Company